Post-Operative Recovery and Pain Relief

Springer

London
Berlin
Heidelberg
New York
Barcelona
Budapest
Hong Kong
Milan
Paris
Santa Clara
Singapore
Tokyo

R. Eltringham, W. Casey and M. Durkin

Post-Operative Recovery and Pain Relief

With 43 Figures

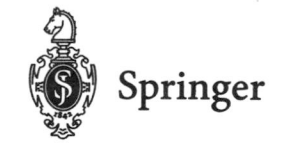 Springer

Roger J. Eltringham, MB, ChB, FRCA
Michael Durkin, MBBS, FRCA
William F. Casey, MB, ChB, FRCA, MA

Department of Anaesthesia, Gloucestershire Royal Hospital,
Gloucester GL1 3NN, UK

ISBN 3-540-76078-4 Springer-Verlag Berlin Heidelberg New York

British Library Cataloguing in Publication Data
Eltringham, Roger
  Post-operative recovery and pain relief
  1. Postoperative care   2. Analgesia
  I. Title   II. Durkin, Michael   III. Casey, William Francis
  617.9'19
ISBN 3540760784

Library of Congress Cataloging-in-Publication Data
Eltringham, Roger, 1939–
  Post-operative recovery and pain relief / R. Eltringham, W. Casey,
and M. Durkin.
     p.   cm.
  Rev. ed. of: Post-anaesthetic recovery / Roger Eltringham ... [et
al.]. 2nd ed. 1989.
  Includes bibliographical references and index.
  ISBN 3-540-76078-4 (pbk. : alk. paper)
  1. Postoperative care.   2. Postoperative pain.   3. Post anesthesia
nursing.   I. Casey, W. (William), 1949-   .   II. Durkin, Michael.
III. Post-anaesthetic recovery.   IV. Title.
  [DNLM: 1. Postanesthesia Nursing.   2. Recovery Room--nurses'
instruction.   3. Postoperative Care--nurses' instruction.
4. Postoperative Complications--prevention & control--nurses'
instruction.   5. Pain, postoperative--therapy--nurses' instruction.
WY 154 E51pa 1997]
RD51.E58   1997
617'.919--dc21
DNLM/DLC   97–14221
for Library of Congress   CIP

Typeset by Richard Powell Editorial & Production Services, Basingstoke, Hants RG22 4TX
Printed and bound at the Athenæum Press Ltd., Gateshead, Tyne & Wear
28/3830-543210   Printed on acid-free paper

Preface

Recent advances in anaesthesia and monitoring have enabled patients who, a few years ago, would have been considered unfit for surgery, now to undergo increasingly complex and lengthy operations in safety.

However, if the good work done by anaesthetists and surgeons in the operating theatre is not to be in vain, high standards of monitoring and patient care must be continued into the critical early post-operative phase when patients are recovering from the immediate effects of their anaesthetic and surgery, and before they are fit to return to general wards. The Medical Defence Societies, the Royal Colleges and a series of reports from the National Confidential Enquiry into Perioperative Deaths have all stressed the vital importance of having appropriate recovery facilities whenever and wherever surgery is performed.

Recovery from anaesthesia may be accompanied by a variety of dangerous and potentially fatal complications, many of which can be avoided by the detection of early warning signs and the institution of appropriate therapy before an irretrievable situation is reached.

This book describes the major problems that may be encountered and suggests how they may be avoided by careful monitoring, vigilant nursing and sound organisation. The behaviour of patients during recovery is influenced by their pre-operative medical condition, by drugs they may receive both pre- and intra-operatively and by the nature of the surgery they have undergone. Sections of the book devoted to each of these areas have been extensively revised to ensure they reflect current best practice.

The section on pain management and regional anaesthesia has been expanded with discussion of patient-controlled analgesia (PCA), continuous epidural narcotic and local anaesthetic infusions, and pleural blockade. We are delighted to have been joined by Dr Jane Brown, one of our consultant anaesthetist colleagues, who has re-written the chapter on Day Surgery to emphasise its ever-increasing importance.

Sue Andrewes, who made immense contributions to the first two editions of this book, is no longer in clinical practice and has decided not to contribute to this edition. We wish to acknowledge that, without her skill and assistance, this book would never have appeared and we wish her and her husband well in their retirement.

We hope that this book will continue to provide a readily available source of practical information not only to nursing staff working in operating theatres and post-operative care units, but also to those working in surgical units, as well as house officers (residents) and junior anaesthetists.

Gloucester, 1997   Roger J. Eltringham
                                                     Michael A. Durkin
                                                     William F. Casey

Contents

Chapter 1
THE ROLE OF THE RECOVERY ROOM

INTRODUCTION

The Association of Anaesthetists of Great Britain and Ireland define the recovery room as "an area to which patients are admitted from an operating room, where they remain until consciousness is regained and ventilation and circulation are stable".

In successive reports, the National Confidential Enquiry into Perioperative Deaths (NCEPOD) has stressed the importance of the recovery room in reducing post-operative morbidity and mortality. In the most recent report (NCEPOD 1992/93), "the provision of a fully staffed and equipped recovery room wherever and whenever patients are to recover from general and regional anaesthesia" is described as the level of modern good practice to which all clinicians should aspire.

Anaesthetists are responsible for the well-being of their patients into the post-operative period. If they are unable to remain with their patients until they are fully recovered, care must only be transferred to staff who are specially trained in recovery procedures. The Medical Defence Union advise that, even if it means holding up the operating list, anaesthetists should not hand over a patient until a competent person is available to take over, and that person declares himself happy to do so. To emphasise the importance of vigilance during the recovery period, there is an increasing tendency, both in the USA and in Europe, to rename recovery rooms as post-anaesthesia care units (PACUs).

DESIGNING A POST-ANAESTHESIA CARE UNIT

The post-anaesthesia care unit should be placed as close to the operating theatres as possible to minimise the risks involved in moving potentially un-stable patients. Although the PACU is often contiguous with the theatre reception ward, the two areas should be kept separate. The reception ward is used as a holding area for patients. It should be quiet so as to allow premedicated patients to wait without undue stress while essential checks are made. Ideally, there should be a separate reception area for children to allow them to be accompanied by their parents.

The ideal number of recovery bays will depend on the number of theatres being served and the type of surgery being undertaken. On average, 1.5 bays per theatre is sufficient, but if theatre throughput is rapid, as in day-surgery units, more will be needed.

The recommended floor area for a standard bay is $9.3\,m^2$ $(100\,ft^2)$ although some larger bays $(18.6\,m^2$ or $200\,ft^2)$ are necessary for patients who may require temporary ventilation or complex monitoring. All bays should have pipeline outlets for oxygen and suction, and some should, in addition, have piped nitrous oxide and respirable air. There should be at least six 13-amp power outlets per bay. It is a distinct advantage to be able to draw curtains around each bay.

The temperature of the PACU should be maintained at approximately 21–22°C with a relative humidity of 38–45%. As patients will continue to exhale volatile anaesthetic agents, there should be a minimum of 15 air changes per hour to minimise pollution. In order to comply with the Control of Substances Hazardous to Health (COSHH) regulations, the efficiency of the ventilation system should be checked at regular intervals by the hospital engineering staff.

Artificial lighting should approximate to the daylight spectrum with a colour temperature of approximately 4000 K. In addition, mobile light sources should be available as they may be needed if demanding procedures are to be undertaken. Care must always to taken to ensure that recovering patients are not dazzled by excessively bright overhead lighting. Many consider it a considerable advantage for there to be windows in the PACU so that there is a source of natural light.

Adequate numbers of sinks, clinical waste containers, telephones and storage space should be available.

AN EFFECTIVE EMERGENCY CALL SYSTEM MUST BE IN PLACE AND ALL STAFF MUST BE FAMILIAR WITH ITS OPERATION.

EQUIPMENT

The equipment needed for an efficiently run PACU can be considered to be as follows:

1. The patient's trolley or bed.
2. Equipment needed at every bay.
3. Cardiorespiratory equipment.
4. Paediatric equipment.
5. Miscellaneous equipment.
6. Drugs and fluids.

Most patients will be taken to the PACU on an operating-theatre trolley. It should have the following characteristics:

(a) An oxygen cylinder of adequate capacity with key, gauge, flowmeter, tubing, suitable oxygen masks and a T-piece attachment for use with laryngeal-mask airways.

(b) Rapid availability of head-down tilt operated from the head end.
(c) Comfortable and easily cleaned mattress.
(d) Adjustable cot side.
(e) Adjustable back rest.
(f) Locking wheels on steerable castors.
(g) Mounting sites for infusion poles.
(h) Tray for notes, X-rays and ancillary equipment such as suction apparatus.

If a hospital bed is used, it should have the same characteristics as a trolley. In addition, it should be height adjustable and have a removable bed head.

Equipment Required at Each Recovery Bay

(a) Oxygen outlet with twin flowmeters: one for use with a disposable oxygen mask or T-piece attachment; the second for use with a Mapleson C circuit or self-inflating Ambu bag.
(b) A variety of oxygen face masks – both fixed and variable performance.
(c) A pulse oximeter.
(d) A suction unit with a supply of differently sized flexible-suction and Yankauer catheters.
(e) Automatic non-invasive blood-pressure measuring equipment or sphygmo-manometer and stethoscope. A full range of cuff sizes should be readily available.
(f) ECG monitor.
(g) Boxes of disposable gloves.
(h) A sharps disposal box.
(i) Separate bins for contaminated reusable and disposable equipment.
(j) Vomit bowl and tissues.
(k) Suitable shelving for storing the above and a writing shelf for holding patients' notes and recovery-room charts.

Additional equipment required in every PACU is as follows:

Cardiorespiratory Equipment

(a) Anaesthetic machine.
(b) Appropriate ventilator with disconnection alarms.
(c) Full selection of oral and nasopharyngeal airways.*
(d) Full range of laryngeal mask airways (LMAs).*
(e) Full range of endotracheal tubes and appropriate intubation equipment (a

---

*This equipment could sensibly all be stored on a single "difficult intubation trolley" that could be moved to an anaesthetic room or operating room if necessary.

range of laryngoscopes and different-sized blades including polio and McCoy blades, gum elastic bougies, stylets, Magill forceps, fibre-optic intubating laryngoscope, etc).*

(f) Crico-thyroid puncture set.*

(g) Bronchoscopes (rigid and fibre optic).*

(h) Jet ventilator.*

(i) Wright's respirometer.*

(j) Infusion sets and a range of intravenous cannulae including central venous and arterial lines.

(k) A range of intravenous fluids, both crystalloid and colloid.

(l) Pressure infusion bags and blood warmers.

(m) Cardiac defibrillator.

(n) Temporary pacing electrodes.

(o) Chest drain set.

(p) Appropriate portable monitoring equipment (ECG, invasive and non-invasive blood-pressure monitors, oximeter and capnograph) to facilitate the safe transfer of patients to intensive care or high-dependency units, or to other hospitals.*

Paediatric Equipment

In general hospitals, where relatively small numbers of young children may be anaesthetised, it is appropriate to have a trolley with a full range of paediatric resuscitation and monitoring equipment that can be rapidly moved between the operating theatres and the PACU.

Miscellaneous Equipment

(a) Thermometers (oral, rectal and low reading).

(b) Warming equipment (hot-air blowers and insulating blankets, infra-red heaters).

(c) Electric blankets for pre-heating beds.

(d) Fans and equipment for managing hyperthermia.

(e) Peripheral nerve stimulators.

(f) Appropriate storage cupboards for drugs, including controlled drugs.

(g) Drug storage fridge.

(h) X-ray viewing boxes.

(i) White boards and marker pens.

(j) Syringes, needles, blood and specimen bottles, laboratory request forms, etc.

(k) Urine and stoma bags, and associated equipment.

---

*This equipment could sensibly all be stored on a single "difficult intubation trolley" that could be moved to an anaesthetic room or operating room if necessary.

(l)   Suitable storage space for pillows, blankets, etc.

(m) Wedge for resuscitating pregnant woman.

Drugs and Intravenous Fluids

An appropriate range of drugs for routine and emergency use must be immediately available. Emergencies to be considered include cardio-respiratory arrest, anaphylaxis and malignant hyperthermia.

Commonly used crystalloid and colloid solutions should be immediately available and there should be easy access to a blood-storage fridge.

SAFETY

Pollution

Patients will exhale nitrous oxide and volatile anaesthetic agents for some time after the end of their anaesthetic. Concern has been expressed about the health risks posed to staff by constant exposure to low concentrations of these drugs. Nitrous oxide and the newer relatively insoluble volatile agents (isoflurane, desflurane and sevoflurane) are rapidly eliminated by the patient, and if the PACU has the recommended 15 air changes per hour, these agents will not represent a significant health hazard.

Blood-borne Infections

Attention has been focused on the dangers staff face from blood-borne infections by the spread of AIDS caused by the HIV viruses. However, the hepatitis B and C viruses pose a much greater threat to medical and nursing staff. Up to 0.5% of the population of western Europe, north America and Australia are asymptomatic carriers of the hepatitis B virus, and consequently, many hundreds of such patient/carriers will pass through every PACU annually. It is therefore recommended that "universal precautions" are practised; that is, all patients are assumed to be potentially infectious and are treated as such. No special additional precautions are then needed for patients who are known to be HIV or hepatitis B or C positive.

The hepatitis viruses are highly infectious; HIV is markedly less so. They are all spread by contamination with blood and other body fluids such as saliva, urine and vaginal secretions. Intact skin is an effective barrier to the viruses but they can enter the circulation through cuts, abrasions and eczematous skin, as well as by needle-stick injuries. Numerous sets of guidelines have been produced to advise staff on how to minimise the risk of contamination. Common recommendations are:

(a) Needles must not be resheathed. Needles, syringes with needles attached and other sharps such as scalpels should not be handed from one person to another. They should be placed in a tray and then picked up.

(b) All needles and other sharps should be disposed of in appropriate, tough disposable bins. These should not be over-filled.

(c) Should a needle-stick injury occur or a cut or abrasion become contaminated with blood, bleeding should be encouraged and the skin washed with soap and water. A record of the incident should be made and the Occupational Health department contacted.

(d) All cuts and abrasions should be covered with waterproof dressings. If lesions are extensive, as is sometimes the case with eczema, gloves should be worn at all times.

(e) Gloves should be worn for venepuncture, setting up intravenous infusions, and inserting and removing airways and endotracheal tubes. Where substantial blood spillage may occur, as when inserting arterial or central venous lines, consideration should be given to wearing a plastic apron, and mask and eye protection.

(f) HIV and hepatitis viruses are not airborne but breathing systems can be contaminated by droplet spray. Filters placed between the patient and the anaesthetic circuit can prevent such droplet contamination.

(g) Equipment likely to become contaminated, should, as far as is practical, be disposable after single use. When this is not possible, it should be autoclaved or washed with soap and water and then immersed in freshly prepared glutaraldehyde for three hours. Floors and other surfaces should be washed with freshly prepared 1% hypochlorite solution.

Hepatitis B is an entirely preventable disease since safe and effective vaccines are available. All at-risk staff should be actively immunised against Hepatitis B and have their antibody status confirmed by testing, as 5% do not sero-convert after a standard immunisation schedule.

STAFFING

Modern anaesthesia and surgery enable increasingly complex procedures to be undertaken successfully. In its turn, this exposes the patient to new risks and demands greater knowledge and skill on the part of medical and nursing staff. All who work in the PACU must be trained to the highest professional standard so that they can provide optimal care immediately, without waiting for outside assistance, should a life-threatening emergency arise.

Although a PACU will be staffed by personnel of varying grades and seniority, all must have a basic understanding of relevant anatomy, physiology and pharmacology, as well as the practical skills needed to maintain the airway and circulation, and undertake cardiopulmonary resuscitation. Staff need to be totally familiar with the monitoring and resuscitation equipment they use, as well as having the nursing skills to care for patients who have undergone a spectrum of surgical procedures. They also need the communication skills, both verbal and non-verbal, to assist parents or carers who wish to be present in the

PACU when their child is recovering from anaesthesia and surgery.

As recovery is not always trouble free, and life-threatening complications can develop very quickly, there should be a one to one staff to patient ratio at all times. The Medical Defence Union advises anaesthetists that "even if it means holding up the operating list, do not hand over the patient until a competent person is available to take over and that person declares himself happy to do so". If emergency surgery is undertaken at night or during weekends, the National Confidential Enquiry into Perioperative Deaths (1990) recommends that an appropriately staffed PACU is essential.

CONTINUING EDUCATION AND TRAINING

All staff should participate in regular in-service training to ensure that their knowledge and skills are maintained and that they are aware of new developments in surgery and anaesthesia. Nurses are, quite rightly, increasingly undertaking tasks that were historically the preserve of doctors. After training and in accordance with local protocols, nurses working in PACUs may:

(a) Administer drugs intravenously.
(b) Top up established epidurals.
(c) Prepare and connect patient-controlled analgesia equipment.
(d) Perform defibrillation.

Time should be allocated for the work of the PACU to be audited systematically, and deficiencies identified and corrected. Critical incidents, which could have led to injury to patients if remedial action had not been taken, should be recorded and steps to prevent them recurring should be implemented.

There is considerable merit in allowing PACU staff to spend time on a regular basis as anaesthetists' assistants in the induction room and in the operating theatre, and to work in the High Dependency and Intensive Care Units. Such rotations are not only of educational value but can also enable staff to gain additional skills, and thus enable them to work in these areas if there are staff shortages or sudden increases in demands for extra skilled staff.

In the United Kingdom, post-basic courses in anaesthetic (ENB 182) and operating department (ENB 183) nursing provide satisfactory training. Operating Department Assistants (ODAs) can obtain City and Guilds Certificate 752 which confirms basic knowledge of anaesthetic, theatre and recovery skills. The National Vocational Qualification (NVQ) in Operating Department Practice, at level 3, ensures knowledge of, and competence in, the skills necessary to care for patients recovering from anaesthesia and surgery, with the exception of the administration of drugs. This skill may be acquired and certified locally.

In the Republic of Ireland, there are no ODAs, and care and assistance are provided by locally trained nurses. The Bord Antranais (Irish Nursing Board) runs full-time, 27-week-long, postgraduate courses in anaesthetic nursing.

POLICIES AND PROTOCOLS

All units should have policies relating to the admission, monitoring and discharge of patients from the PACU. Staff should be familiar with these policies and they should be regularly reviewed and, if necessary, revised. National protocols for cardiopulmonary resuscitation should be followed and local protocols for the management of complications, such as malignant hyperthermia, should be devised. Likewise, protocols for demanding and potentially hazardous procedures, such as the intravenous administration of drugs and the management of epidural infusions, should be prepared and followed.

RECOVERY STAFF SHOULD KNOW PRECISELY HOW TO SUMMON HELP IN THE CASE OF AN EMERGENCY.

References and Bibliography

The Report of the National Confidential Enquiry into Perioperative Deaths (1990).
The Report of the National Confidential Enquiry into Perioperative Deaths (1991/92).
The Report of the National Confidential Enquiry into Perioperative Deaths (1992/93).
Aids and Hepatitis B: Guidelines for Anaesthetists (1988). Association of Anaesthetists.
Immediate Postanaesthetic Recovery (1993). Association of Anaesthetists.
Risk Management in Day Unit Surgery (1992). Medical Defence Union.
Risk Management in Anaesthesia (1991). Medical Defence Union.
Hospital Building Note (1975). Department of Health and Social Security.
Children First. A Study of Hospital Services (1993). Audit Commission, HMSO, London.
Control of Substances Hazardous to Health. Guidance for the Initial Assessment in Hospitals (1989). Department of Health.

Chapter 2
NORMAL RECOVERY

PHYSIOLOGY OF THE ELIMINATION OF DRUGS USED DURING ANAESTHESIA

Patients recover from anaesthesia as the agents given to maintain anaesthesia are either excreted or metabolised.

Volatile Agents

These are largely excreted unchanged by the lungs. The more soluble the agent the slower is the rate of elimination. Thus recovery from a soluble agent such as ether (blood gas solubility 12) is prolonged, while recovery from less soluble agents such as desflurane (0.4) and sevoflurane (0.6) is more rapid. However, a significant percentage of halothane (over 20%) is metabolised in the liver and then excreted in the urine. Lesser amounts of enflurane (2%), isoflurane (0.2%) and desflurane (0.02%) are also metabolised.

Intravenous Induction Agents

Their duration of action is largely determined by their rates of distribution and metabolism. These are rapid in the case of propofol and etomidate, after which recovery is correspondingly fast, but slower with thiopentone. Repeated doses of thiopentone are followed by prolonged drowsiness, and dosages should be reduced in the presence of liver disease and in the elderly. Ketamine is characterised by slower distribution and metabolism, and a prolonged recovery period can be expected.

Suxamethonium

This is rapidly metabolised by pseudo-cholinesterase in the blood. Recovery from suxamethonium usually occurs within 3–5 minutes. Occasionally, a patient may lack pseudo-cholinesterase. Suxamethonium is then metabolised more slowly in the liver. This may take several hours. During that time, the patient should be ventilated and sedated. Subsequently, the patient's general practitioner should be informed and close relatives should be screened to determine if they too lack the relevant enzyme.

Non-depolarising Muscle Relaxants

These normally have their action reversed by an anticholinesterase (neostigmine) at the end of the surgical procedure. However, atracurium and vecuronium are shorter acting and do not always need formal reversal. Vecuronium is metabolised in the liver while atracurium undergoes Hoffman degradation, i.e. it spontaneously breaks down at body temperature and pH. Mivacurium has an even shorter duration of action and is metabolised by plasma cholinesterase.

Analgesics

Analgesics given pre-operatively or intra-operatively should preferably still be active so that patients do not recover consciousness to find themselves in severe pain.

To understand the reversal of an anaesthetic, when volatile agents have been used, is to recognise that the elimination pathway is similar to that of its uptake. The same physiological rules control the blood–gas partition coefficient and the solubility rating. At their withdrawal the anaesthetic gases, with their higher partial pressure in the venous blood carried by the pulmonary artery, diffuse across to the lower pressure of the alveolar space. A gas of low solubility in blood (e.g. nitrous oxide) will rapidly transfer to the alveolar space. The rate of fall of the alveolar concentration is in proportion to the patient's ventilatory performance.

We will therefore be seeing the importance of output controlled by blood gas solubility, venous/alveolar partial pressure changes, and cardiac and respiratory performance. However, at the time of elimination, important factors adversely affect the smooth dispersal of the gases. The high concentrations of nitrous oxide which easily pass across the alveolar space displace the oxygen of the inspired atmospheric air in the lungs. This is called *diffusion hypoxaemia*, the Fink effect.

Cardiac output may have become reduced by myocardial depression caused by anaesthetic drugs, and respiratory function can be reduced if any central depression of the brain's respiratory centre exists. This central depression may also obtain when major analgesic drugs have been used concurrently with the general anaesthetic.

First a yardstick should be established by which to assess the patient's normal progress at the post-anaesthetic recovery time. The variable effects of an anaesthetic will then more easily be noted.

PROGRESS OF NORMAL RECOVERY

Depth of anaesthesia is determined by physical signs and is classically divided into stages I–IV as described by Guedel (1933).

During the recovery from anaesthesia the stages are seen in the reverse order (Table 2.1).

Table 2.1. Observations in the reversing stages of anaesthesia

Observations	Stage 3 Surgical anaesthesia	Stage 2 Excitement	Stage 1 Analgesia	Normal
Muscle tone		Tense or struggling		
Respirations Intercostal / Diaphragmatic				
Conscious level	Unconscious		Rousable	Conscious Cooperates Comprehends
Blood pressure, systolic			Fluctuating	Normal readings

Stage IV: Medullary Paralysis

This is characterised by respiratory arrest and occurs as a result of an overdose of anaesthetic agents. This must be reversed at once and is not seen during the recovery period.

Stage III: The Stage of Surgical Anaesthesia

During emergence from this stage, which is divided into four planes, there is a gradual return of muscle tone and reflexes (Table 2.2, *overleaf*). The purely diaphragmatic breathing seen in the deeper planes is replaced by the normal pattern of breathing as intercostal tone returns.

Stage II: The Stage of Excitement

During this stage the patient may struggle and make uncoordinated movements. Reflexes have returned and vomiting may occur. Difficulties may be encountered in extending a patient's forearm when making a blood-pressure measurement at this time.

Stage I: The Stage of Analgesia

Analgesia is wearing off and the patient gradually regains consciousness. Female patients are liable to become tearful and male patients may be aggressive or amorous. Fortunately there is seldom any recollection of this.

Table 2.2. The returning reflexes

Reflexes	Stage 3 Surgical anaesthesia	Stage 2 Excitement	Stage 1 Analgesia	Normal
Swallowing Vomiting Laryngeal (cords) Coughing				
Bite reflex				
Eyelash reflex Eyelid reflex				
Secretion of tears				

Although progress of recovery may be assessed within the framework, it must be emphasised that many factors influence the return of consciousness, e.g. medical history, premedication and anaesthetic technique (see Chapter 6), so that a knowledge of these is essential for intelligent recovery nursing.

CARE-PLAN NURSING

The type of nursing required for the rapid turnover of high-dependency short-stay patients needs careful planning. No matter how many patients are seen nor how routine the procedure, each patient must be treated as an individual with particular needs. These needs will be related not only to the operation and the anaesthetic but also to a large extent to the patient's social and medical history. To nurse solely with information concerning the operative and anaesthetic procedure is to nurse the patient with some degree of ignorance. It is neither the time nor the place to be searching through the medical notes for information when the patient has already been admitted to the recovery unit.

To enable recovery staff to anticipate the patient's requirements, basic information should be available on each patient before his arrival from the operating theatre. It should be supplied either by the ward staff or, if it is practical, by the recovery staff following a pre-operative visit to the patient on the ward. This account of the patient will be recorded as a pre-operative picture of his needs and be transferred to the chart in the PACU room. Data processing facilities should, if possible, be made available for the unit.

The information required on each patient before operation should include:

1. Name and age, unit number (and marital status in the case of females) on identification band.
2. Medical history of significance, with special reference to respiratory and cardiovascular systems with blood pressure and pulse rate.
3. Drug therapy.
4. Allergies.
5. Skin state and general colour.
6. Dental state.
7. Hearing and vision problems.
8. Command of English (a list of useful phrases in other languages is given in Appendix B).
9. Emotional state.
10. Belongings sent with patient, e.g. hearing aid, spectacles, toys.
11. Weight.
12. Haemoglobin and other biochemical results.

The patient's identification wrist band must be checked for its accuracy. As well as the site of the proposed operation, the left or right side should be marked.

RECEPTION OF THE PATIENT

When the patient arrives, the recovery nurse should receive a full report from the anaesthetist, which should include:

1. The patient's name.
2. The surgical procedure performed and the name of the surgeon.
3. The anaesthetic technique used and its duration.
4. The blood loss and intraoperative fluid replacement.
5. The final monitoring record.
6. Any complications encountered during anaesthesia.
7. The number and type of drains or catheters.
8. The presence of packs remaining *in situ*.
9. The post-anaesthetic requirements for:
    (a) the positioning of the patient.
    (b) oxygen therapy.
    (c) intravenous fluid.
    (d) drug therapy.

Before the recovery staff take over the responsibility of the care of the patient they must satisfy themselves that:

1. The breathing is regular and unobstructed.
2. A good colour is being maintained.
3. The pulse is palpable and regular.

If they are concerned about any of these vital considerations, they should inform the anaesthetist immediately.

BASIC NURSING POSITION AND SAFETY

As with a tiny baby, the many needs of the unconscious patient should be anticipated. The nursing approach should be that of "positive protective care" and not just "tender loving care".

On arrival in the recovery unit:

1. The nurse should check that the patient is on the trolley the correct way round, i.e. so the patient can be tilted head down (Trendelenburg position) if necessary.
2. The nurse should station herself at the patient's head with all the necessary equipment within arms' reach.
3. The brakes should be applied to the trolley or bed.
4. The patient will normally be nursed on the side, and the position should be made secure with a supporting back pillow (see Figure 2.1). It is advisable for the anaesthetist to turn the patient on to his side electively and in a controlled manner, with assistance, before leaving the operating room rather than to risk the possibility of a nurse struggling to achieve this single-handedly later on in an emergency.
5. The side rails should be raised throughout the patient's recovery time.

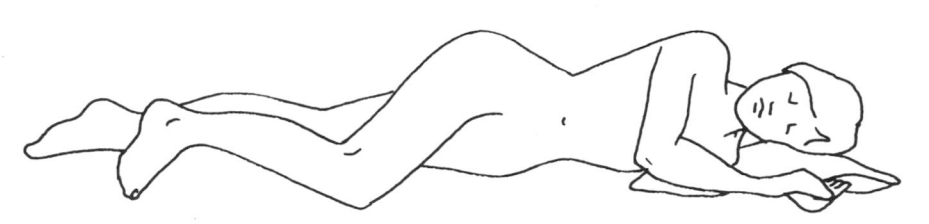

Figure 2.1 The normal recovery position

ROUTINE OBSERVATIONS

As soon as the patient has been transferred to the care of the recovery staff, they must assume full responsibility for his well-being until all the criteria for discharge have been met (see page 42) and the patient is returned to the care of the ward staff.

The patient is kept under continuous observation and the findings recorded at least every 15 minutes. These recordings should not be seen in isolation but as a part of a trend so that potential problems can be anticipated and corrected before a dangerous and possibly irreversible situation is allowed to develop.

The order of taking observations is as follows:

1. Colour.
2. Respiratory function.
3. Cardiovascular function.
4. Level of consciousness.
5. Blood.

Following the baseline recordings on admission, an absolute minimum of two subsequent recordings are made at 15-minute intervals (i.e. for ½ hour). If complications arise or if medications or units of blood are given, recordings may be required more frequently and a further period of observation of at least 30 minutes will be required.

The temperature is not taken routinely on all patients. However, following prolonged surgery, large transfusions or if the temperature seems abnormal, it is recorded and the patient is kept in recovery until gross deviations have been corrected.

Inspections should be made of the wound dressing, the character and amounts of drainage and the diathermy site for evidence of burns.

ASSESSMENT OF COLOUR

The routine use of oximetry is recommended for all patients recovering from anaesthesia as this gives an early warning of reduced oxygenation. However, if this is unavailable, reliance must be placed on continuing clinical observation.

With normal cardiovascular and respiratory function a supply of well-oxygenated blood is delivered to the tissues, which appear pink. If the blood is not being adequately oxygenated or the blood supply to the tissues is impaired, the normal pink appearance is replaced by cyanosis or pallor. If well-perfused areas, such as the lips, appear cyanosed, this indicates either respiratory or cardiac dysfunction and immediate attention must be given to these systems. In dark-skinned patients an examination of the inside of the mouth or the conjunctival vessels will provide the same information.

Peripheral and Central Cyanosis

These two signs may be assessed in the following way. Peripheral cyanosis is seen at the fingers, toes and tip of the nose. It signifies a low cardiac output and can also be seen with low systolic blood pressure caused by hypovolaemia. Central cyanosis, seen at the lips, tongue and conjunctiva, is a sign of impaired gas exchange between the alveoli and the pulmonary capillaries. In the recovery period the most usual cause is hypoventilation or lung ventilation/perfusion imbalance. A practical method to differentiate between the two states is to massage the cyanotic skin, whereupon peripheral cyanosis will disappear; central cyanosis will not.

ASSESSMENT OF RESPIRATORY FUNCTION

Recovery staff must observe respiratory performance critically throughout the recovery period and recognise any departure from normal.

In normal breathing:

1. The patient's colour is satisfactory. There is no cyanosis of well-perfused areas.
2. The movement of warm expired air can be felt by placing the hand in front of the mouth or nose.
3. The chest and abdomen rise together with inspiration. The chest should not retract as the abdomen rises; this would produce a rocking or see-saw motion.
4. The breathing pattern is regular with a rate between 12 and 24 per minute in adults.
5. Breathing is silent. There should be no stertorous (snoring), no stridor and no gurgling sound from the pharynx, and there should be no wheezing.
6. Breathing appears effortless. The accessory muscles of respiration (sterno-mastoids and scalenes) should not be in use and the head should not retract with inspiration. The thyroid cartilage and upper trachea should not be drawn down during inspiration (tracheal tug). There should be no flaring of the nostrils on inspiration.

Any departure from the signs of normal breathing listed above must receive immediate attention since rapid deterioration in the patient's condition may follow (see Chapter 4).

ASSESSMENT OF CARDIOVASCULAR FUNCTION

When cardiovascular function is normal:

1. The tissues are well perfused.
2. The pulses are easily palpable and regular.
3. The heart rate and blood pressure approximate to normal pre-operative values.

Tissue Perfusion

Tissue perfusion is estimated by examination of the skin. This should be warm, pink and dry. There should be no pallor or cyanosis. Poor peripheral perfusion is indicated by cold pale extremities and a weak thready pulse. The nail beds provide a useful site for inspection. With variable lighting conditions a comparison of the attendant's own nail bed can serve as a useful reference. There should be a rapid return of colour following digital compression of the nail bed.

Pulse Measurement

The pulse may be taken at the following sites:

1. The radial artery at the wrist (in paediatric patients the brachial artery may be easier to feel).
2. The temporal artery (Figure 2.2).
3. The facial artery as it crosses the border of the mandible in front of the insertion of the masseter muscle. This can conveniently be felt by the ring finger while maintaining the patient's airway (Figure 2.3, *overleaf*).
4. If these pulses cannot be felt, the carotid artery must be sought (Figure 2.4, *overleaf*) so as to confirm cardiac function.

In addition to the above, confirmation of the pulse at the following sites may be useful after vascular or orthopaedic surgery:

5. The femoral artery.
6. The popliteal artery.
7. The dorsalis pedis artery.   } (see Figure 2.5, *overleaf*)
8. The posterior tibial artery.

All pulse rates should be counted over a minute and any irregularities noted. If the pulse is weak and difficult to palpate, this should be recorded.

With babies it may be more practical to listen to the heart itself, using the diaphragm of a stethoscope secured over the precordium with light strapping.

Doppler Ultrasonic Recorder

This instrument is of value when assessing blood flow when a pulse is not easily palpated. It will also confirm arterial patency in the limb distal to vascular surgical sites.

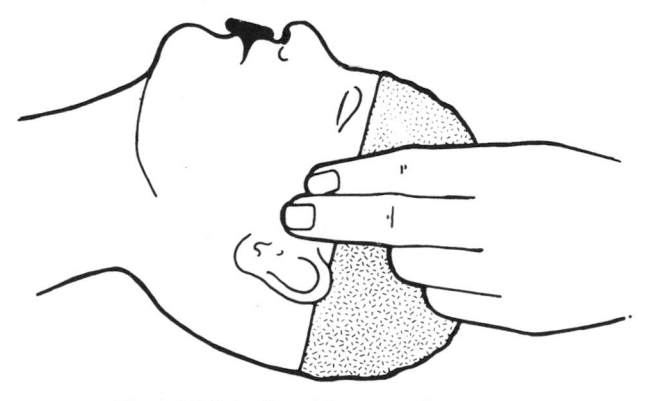

Figure 2.2 Palpation of the temporal artery

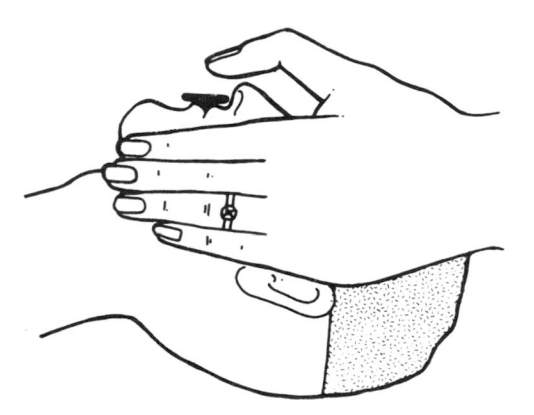

Figure 2.3 Palpation of the facial artery with ring finger

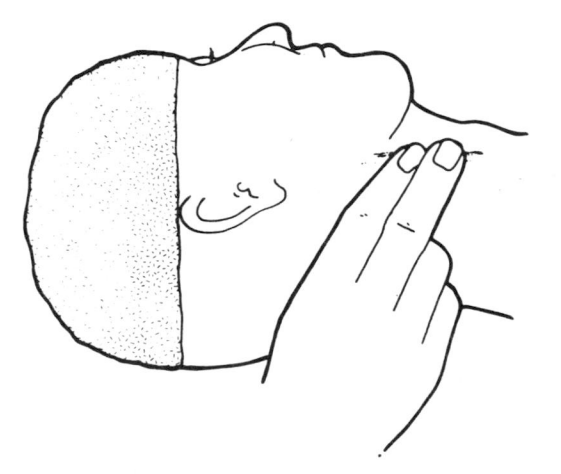

Figure 2.4 Palpation of the carotid artery medial and deep to the sternomastoid muscle

Blood Pressure Measurement

Absolute values of blood pressure are less important than a trend and should be interpreted in relation to the patient's general condition. Any major deviation from normal pre-operative values will require attention (see pages 80–83), particularly if it is accompanied by other cardiovascular abnormalities such as poor peripheral perfusion or changes in heart rate or rhythm.

Sphygmomanometer and Stethoscope

It is important to use the correct size of cuff. With a standard cuff, false high readings are obtained in obese patients and false low readings in thin patients.

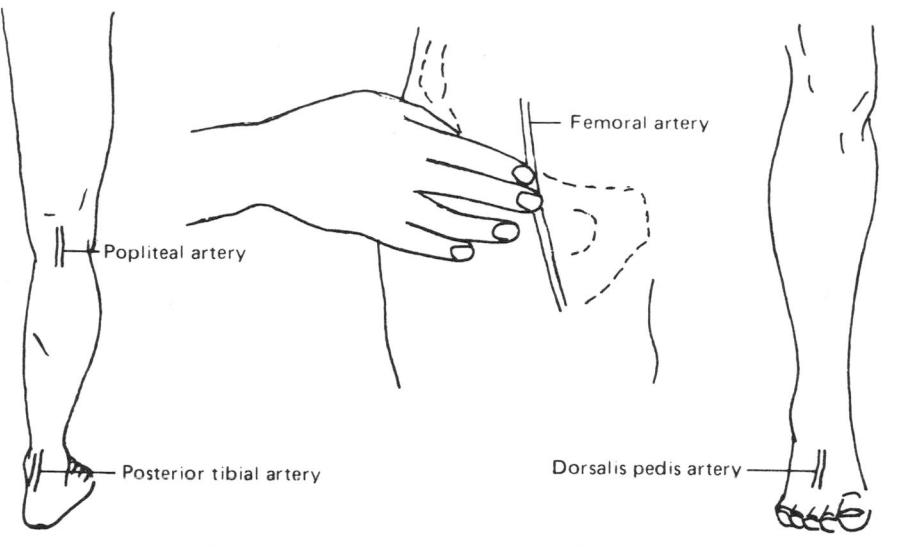

Figure 2.5 Position of the main arteries in the right leg

The width of the cuff bladder should be 20% greater than the arm's diameter (see Table 2.3). The cuff should be immediately deflated after use and removed if used on the same limb receiving an intravenous infusion.

Table 2.3. Width of sphygmomanometer cuff bladder

	Bladder width (cm)	Length (cm)
Thigh	18.5	38.5
Obese	15	38
Adult	12.5	25
Child	8.5	18
Infant	6	12
Neonate	4	7.5

Pulse pressure is the difference between systolic and diastolic blood pressure readings. A difference of less than 40 mmHg may indicate falling cardiac output and is therefore a useful evaluation of the patient's perfusion state.

Oscillotonometer

This is satisfactory only when the patient is anaesthetised. As muscle tone returns, the needle swings with every muscle contraction and accuracy is impaired.

Automatic Blood-pressure Recording

Various types of apparatus are available for automatic measurement and display of blood pressure using an oscillotonometer principle, e.g. the Dinamap®

Accutorr. The frequency of recordings can be adjusted according to the patient's requirements. Although these devices save nursing time, they should not be regarded as an alternative to close observations of the patient.

Direct Arterial Pressure Measurement

During major surgery, blood pressure is sometimes measured directly following insertion of a cannula into the lumen of an artery and the pressure displayed by an aneroid manometer (e.g. the Tycos manometer) or on a monitor screen via a transducer. Direct arterial pressure measurements are often continued post-operatively, and recovery staff should be familiar with the principles involved.

For accurate readings the transducer should be on the same level as the heart and must first be calibrated to zero at this level. To maintain the patency of the lumen the cannula must be flushed with heparinised saline either intermittently by a syringe or, preferably, by continuous infusion. This can be conveniently achieved by attaching a litre bag of sodium chloride 0.9% containing 1000 units of heparin via a giving set to the side arm of a continuous flushing device (e.g. the Intraflo®). To maintain a slow infusion, the heparinised saline is kept at a pressure of about 300 mmHg inside a pressure bag. If the arterial trace becomes damped or if a blood sample is taken from the arterial line it should be flushed with an additional bolus of heparinised saline.

The arterial cannula should be well away from intravenous infusion sites and must be clearly labelled as such, so that injections cannot inadvertently be given intra-arterially.

The cannulation site should not be hidden by dressings but should be protected by a small transparent covering to allow frequent inspection. This is necessary:

(a) To detect impairment of the circulation occurring distally.

(b) To detect haematoma formation.

(c) Because disconnection will lead to severe blood loss.

In the event of (a) or (b) occurring, or if measurements are no longer required, the cannula is removed. This is done using an aseptic technique followed by application of firm digital pressure via a sterile dressing on the cannulation site for a full 5 min. If bleeding continues after this, pressure must be maintained until it has stopped.

Additional information on cardiovascular function can be obtained by the following:

Examination of Venous Filling

The veins should be well filled and neither collapsed nor over-distended. Veins on the forearms and hand are suitable for examination. Neck veins are less useful in the supine position as they are generally distended unless there is severe hypo-volaemia.

ECG Monitoring

The ECG monitor records electrical activity of the heart but yields no information about its mechanical efficiency. It is not required routinely on all patients in the recovery room but can provide useful information on the nature of cardiac irregularities (page 87) or evidence of myocardial ischaemia (page 149). Its use is recommended when there is a history of dysrhythmias or when pre- or intra-operative medications have been used to treat cardiovascular instability. Recovery staff should be able to recognise a normal trace and the common dysrhythmias, and should refer abnormalities for interpretation, especially if accompanied by other evidence of cardiovascular dysfunction.

A full 12-lead record will be required if myocardial infarction or pulmonary embolus are suspected.

Central Venous Pressure (CVP)

This reflects a balance between cardiac output and circulating blood volume and can be measured by placing the tip of a catheter in the superior vena cava, the exact position being confirmed radiologically. Readings can be taken by a simple manometer consisting of a column of fluid connected to an intravenous infusion by a three-way tap (Figure 2.6, *overleaf*), the meniscus fluctuating in time with the respirations. It is important to ensure that the tubing between the manometer and the patient loops well below the cannula site in order to prevent air entering the vein if the CVP reading is sub-atmospheric. Readings may also be taken via a transducer as for arterial pressure readings.

It is important that all readings are taken from the same well-defined anatomical landmark, such as the fourth thoracic interspace in the mid-axillary line. The normal range is 5–15 cm of water although absolute values are of less importance than the trend in response to therapy. In general, high readings suggest fluid overload or cardiac dysfunction while low readings suggest a reduced circulating blood volume.

Pulmonary Capillary Wedge Pressure (PCWP)

In the critically ill patient a discrepancy may exist between the left and right ventricular performance. An indication of left ventricular function can be obtained by use of a balloon-tipped flotation catheter, e.g. the Swan-Ganz catheter.

The simplest type has two lumens; one measures the pressure at the tip and is connected to a pressure transducer, while the other is used to inflate the balloon with air. The catheter is inserted via a central vein into the right atrium, the balloon inflated with a maximum of 2 ml air and the catheter advanced until it wedges in the pulmonary artery. With the balloon inflated the pulmonary capillary wedge pressure is obtained. This reflects left atrial pressure. With the balloon deflated the pulmonary artery pressure is obtained. More sophisticated modifications may also have a proximal lumen opening into the right atrium and a thermistor at the tip for measurements of cardiac output by a thermodilution technique.

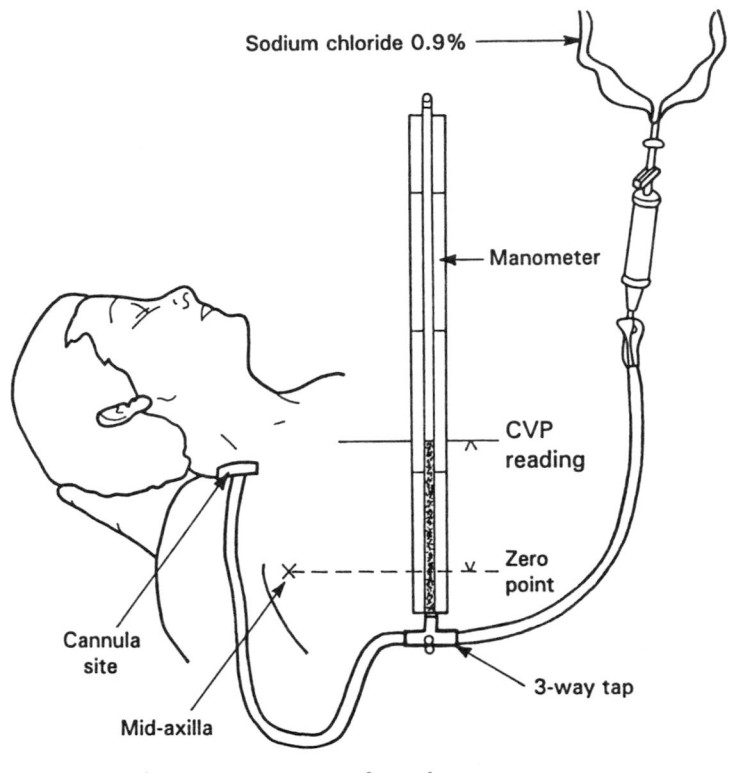

Figure 2.6 Measurement of central venous pressure

When a patient with a Swan-Ganz catheter *in situ* arrives in the recovery room, the transducer is recalibrated, the pressure displayed on a monitor screen and the patency of the lumen maintained by a continuous flushing device.

The recovery staff must be able to:

(a) Identify the various lumens of the catheter.
(b) Recognise the pulmonary artery trace on the monitor screen.
(c) Inflate the balloon with air, identify the wedge trace and record the pressure.
(d) Deflate the balloon when this measurement has been made and ensure that the pulmonary artery trace reappears.

Care must be taken to ensure that the balloon is kept deflated between wedge-pressure measurements, since prolonged wedging will cause pulmonary damage. The catheter tip may spontaneously advance into the wedge position, in which case it must be withdrawn until the pulmonary artery trace reappears.

Only sufficient air to produce a wedge tracing is required when inflating the balloon using a maximum of 2 ml. Over-inflation will cause pulmonary damage and may rupture the balloon.

If recovery staff are asked to remove the catheter it is important that the balloon is, of course, deflated first, so as to avoid damage to the valves of the heart.

Urine Output

Urine output is taken as an index of tissue perfusion in patients with healthy kidneys. An output in excess of 0.5 ml/(kg h) indicates adequate renal perfusion, i.e. 15 ml for a 60 kg patient every half an hour. It is measured in a urine bag following the insertion of a Foley catheter. The bag is emptied and the amount recorded on admitting the patient to the recovery unit. Thereafter measurements should be made every 30 min. The presence of blood in the urine should be noted and the surgeon informed. Small amounts of urine cannot be measured with any accuracy using the graduations of a 1- or 2-litre bag. Drainage systems incorporating small-volume urine meters should be used or readings taken using a 50 ml syringe. The standard tubing from catheter to bag contains 3.5 ml per 10 cm length.

ASSESSMENT OF LEVEL OF CONSCIOUSNESS

As soon as the anaesthetic administration ceases there should be a progressive return of consciousness as the agents are eliminated or metabolised. The level of consciousness is monitored:

1. To ensure that there is steady progress towards full consciousness and that there is no undue prolongation of unconsciousness requiring investigation or treatment.
2. To determine when the patient has regained full consciousness, his protective reflexes have returned and he is able to maintain his own airway.

Elaborate monitoring as used following cerebral trauma is not required. The level of consciousness can be simply estimated by the following:

1. Return of eyelid reflex.
2. Return of bite reflex.
3. Response to moderate stimulation, e.g. gently rubbing the cheek.
4. Ability to obey simple commands, e.g. "open your eyes".
5. Ability to respond to questions, e.g. "have you any pain?"

Hearing is one of the first senses to return following anaesthesia and can be demonstrated by an appropriate response to a simple question, such as "Are you in pain?" or "Can you breathe easily?" Discussion of the patient's operative procedure or prognosis with colleagues should obviously be avoided. The above simple commands enable patients to demonstrate their return to consciousness and their ability to co-operate.

Painful stimulation is not required during routine recovery and should, as a practice, certainly be discouraged. It may be unpleasant for the patient, it may cause bruising and occasionally it provokes a violent response. Nevertheless, such stimulation may be used with discretion as a guide to progress if unconsciousness is unduly prolonged and a coma level assessment is required (page 128).

Observation of the pupils is not routinely used as a guide to progress since many factors affect pupil size. When the anaesthetic agents have been eliminated, normal pupils are equal in size and react to light. Regular examination of the pupils is required after a period of cerebral hypoxia, following neurosurgery or cerebral trauma, or if unconsciousness is prolonged.

Dilation of the pupils (mydriasis) can be caused by:

1. Ganglion-blocking agents used to produce hypotensive anaesthesia.
2. Large doses of atropine.
3. Ether and cyclopropane administration and deep planes of anaesthesia.
4. Mydriatic eye drops, e.g. cyclopentolate, phenylephrine.

Constricted pupils (miosis) can be caused by:

1. Opiate administration.
2. Miotic eye drops, e.g. pilocarpine.

RECOGNITION OF BLOOD LOSS

The patient may continue to lose blood in the post-operative period and evidence of this must be sought by regular inspection of wound dressings, packs, vaginal pad, drainage bottles and bladder irrigation. Continued bleeding must be referred to the surgeon and anaesthetist as further surgery and blood transfusion may be required.

If signs of hypovolaemia develop (hypotension, tachycardia, pallor or sweating) when there is no visible blood loss, internal haemorrhage must be suspected. The patient's girth measurements are seldom helpful as it is now recognised that internal haemorrhage can be extensive without an increase in the abdominal size.

MAINTENANCE OF THE AIRWAY

In the unconscious patient with the chin relaxed, the tongue is liable to fall back and obstruct the airway. To avoid this the head must be extended and the mandible held forwards. This can usually be achieved with one hand. The tips of the fingers are placed under the point of the jaw, which is lifted forwards and upwards so that the expired air can be felt against the palm of the hand (Figure 2.7).

In the overweight patient with a short thick neck it may be impossible to displace the mandible in this way and a two-handed approach is required. The middle fingers of both hands are placed behind the angles of the mandible, which is lifted forwards. The fingers are spread with the forefingers at the tip of the chin, leaving the thumbs to feel the expired are or to hold a face mask (Figure 2.8).

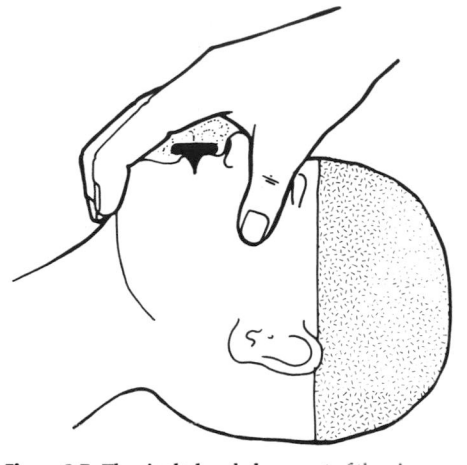

Figure 2.7 The single-handed support of the airway

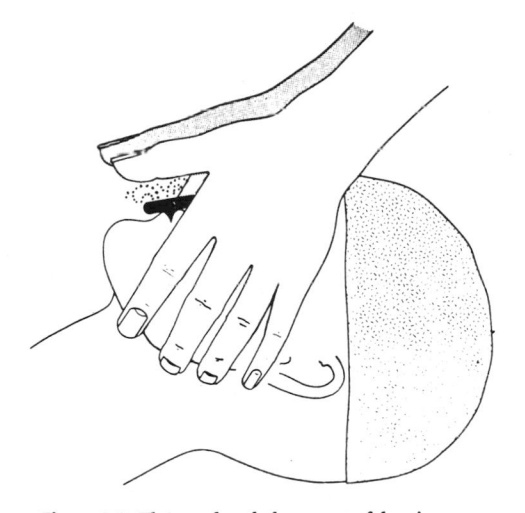

Figure 2.8 The two-handed support of the airway

INSERTION OF OROPHARYNGEAL AIRWAY

An oropharyngeal airway, e.g. the Guedel airway, may be inserted to prevent the tongue falling back and consequently obstructing breathing. Such airways are made of moulded rubber or plastic and come in various sizes:

- Large males   Size 4
- Standard adult males   Size 3
- Adult females   Size 2
- Paediatric range   Sizes 1, 0, 00 and 000

The size should be large enough to go beyond the back of the tongue but should not press on the posterior pharyngeal wall as this may stimulate the gag reflex. A check should be made that the rubber is in good order and that the metal insert is in place.

The airway is first lubricated with gel then introduced upside down and rotated in the vault of the mouth so that it slips down behind the tongue (Figure 2.9). The patient's teeth (or gums in an edentulous patient) should bite down on the metal insert (flanged) end. Patency may be obliterated if the bite takes place on an unreinforced area. It should be checked that the lips do not come between the teeth and the airway as bleeding or swelling may result. It should also be confirmed that the lips do not fold over to obstruct the air entry.

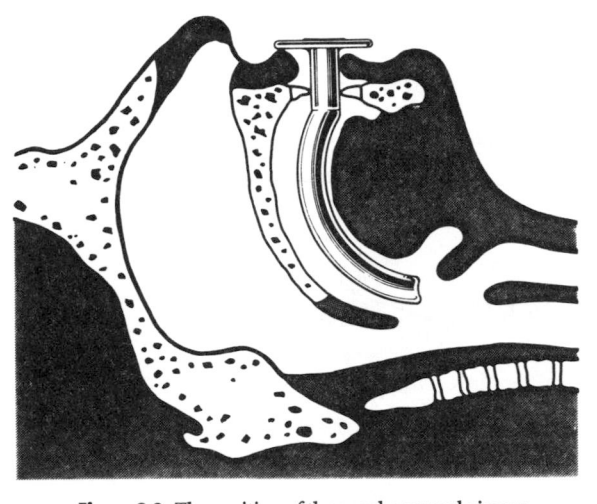

Figure 2.9 The position of the oropharyngeal airway

INSERTION OF NASOPHARYNGEAL AIRWAY

This may be required if:

1. The airway cannot be maintained using a Guedel airway.
2. The jaws are clamped tightly together and it is impossible to insert a Guedel airway.
3. The jaws are wired together following dental or faciomaxillary surgery (see page 124).
4. Dental bridges and crowned or broken teeth are vulnerable to biting on a Guedel airway.
5. There has been surgery to the mouth.

The nasopharyngeal airway consists of a curved tube with a flanged lip at the nasal opening (Figure 2.10). It is manufactured to resist kinking and comes in four sizes of internal diameter 9.0 mm, 8.0 mm, 7.0 mm and 6.0 mm.

To introduce the nasopharyngeal airway it is first lubricated and then inserted with half-rotating movements for its total length. Deviation of the nasal septum may indicate one side for easier insertion. Bleeding may be provoked and a fine suction catheter should be available which will fit inside the tube to clear the pharynx of blood. The introduction of a nasopharyngeal airway is unwise in patients on anticoagulants or with a bleeding disorder.

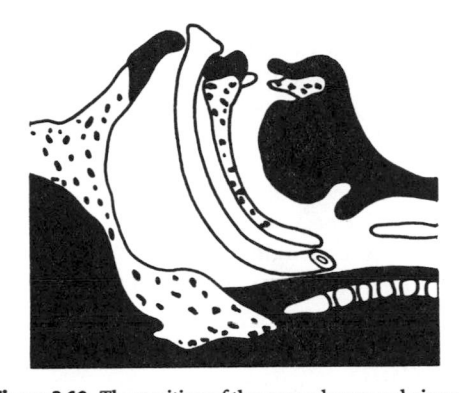

Figure 2.10   The position of the naso-pharyngeal airway

SUCTION OF THE UPPER AIRWAY

Any fluid or foreign material in the mouth or pharynx should be removed by suction as it may:

1. Obstruct the airway.
2. Irritate the larynx and cause laryngeal spasm during the light stages of anaesthesia.
3. Be inhaled into the lungs if the laryngeal reflexes are yet to return.
4. Provoke violent coughing spasms.

The negative pressure (vacuum) setting should be within the range of 100–120 mmHg so that there is no damage to the mucosal surfaces. Suction is indicated if gurgling sounds are heard during respiration, if the airway is obstructed and if there is breath holding or vomiting (see pages 97–99). Suction can be applied by a rigid Yankauer sucker or by a soft catheter. Catheter sizes range from F.G. (French gauge) 6 for neonates up to F.G. 22. The tip of the catheter can be advanced blindly behind the back of the tongue either beside or through the oropharyngeal airway. A catheter size of F.G. 10 may be introduced down a Guedel airway.

After oral or throat surgery, suction should be performed by the anaesthetist under direct vision using a laryngoscope. Blind suction is inadvisable under these circumstances as it may dislodge clots or ligatures. A bowl of water should be available to clear the sucker if it becomes blocked by viscid secretions.

In susceptible patients suction may provoke bradycardia due to vagal stimulation. It may be noted that atropine given at the reversal stage of non-depolarising muscle relaxants will produce tenacious secretions affecting the respiratory tract. Unpleasant dryness of the mouth may be relieved, when the patient is fully arousable, by moistening the mouth with water on a swab. The swab should be mounted on sponge-holding forceps.

CARE OF THE INTUBATED PATIENT

Patients are occasionally admitted to the recovery room with an endotracheal tube in place. Recovery staff must be certain that it is well secured and does not become accidentally dislodged or obstructed by secretions or by kinking. If it is to be retained for more than a short period, humidification will be required as natural humidification provided by the upper airway is bypassed, so that secretions will become viscid and crusting may result. This is especially important in children in whom obstruction may easily occur with the narrower endotracheal tube sizes. Frequent suction down the entire length of the tube is required. Humidified oxygen may be best administered via a T-piece system (page 31).

Endotracheal Suction

Before commencing suction, 100% oxygen is administered and the patient is warned of the procedure even if he does not appear to be conscious. A soft Aeroflo catheter with an occluding port is used and the suction is set at 100–120 mmHg of vacuum. The nurses carrying out the procedure wear gloves for their own protection and to avoid introducing infection. The catheter is passed down the endotracheal tube, ensuring the tip goes beyond the end of the tube; a finger is then placed on the occluding port and the catheter is slowly withdrawn using a rotating movement, after which the oxygen supply is reconnected. The duration of suction should be limited to 5 s. This procedure is repeated using a fresh catheter each time until the trachea is clear.

Extubation

Before extubation is attempted:

1. Adequate spontaneous breathing must be established.
2. Laryngeal and pharyngeal reflexes must be present.
3. 100% oxygen is administered for several minutes.
4. The larynx and pharynx are cleared by suction above the inflated balloon cuff.
5. The tape or strapping securing the tube is released.
6. The patient is on his side and head down if there is a risk of vomiting or re-gurgitation.

An oropharyngeal airway (Guedel) may then be inserted, the endotracheal tube cuff is deflated and the tube removed at the end of an inspiration. The patient must be watched closely in the period immediately following extubation as respiratory difficulties are liable to occur at this time. Of particular importance are laryngeal stridor and laryngeal spasm, which will require immediate attention (page 68).

CARE OF THE PATIENT WITH A LARYNGEAL MASK AIRWAY (LMA)

In contrast to the endotracheal tube, the LMA is well tolerated by the patient emerging from GA and can usually be kept in place until the patient attempts to remove it himself. The cuff is then deflated and the tube is removed with accompanying suction, as necessary. While in place, supplementary oxygen can be administered using a T-piece with a high flow of oxygen (10 l/min). The LMA is not disposable and after removal is cleaned and sent for autoclaving. Because of the gradual deterioration with repeated use, a maximum of 40 insertions is recommended, after which it should be discarded.

THE VENTILATED PATIENT

If adequate spontaneous respiration is not established at the conclusion of surgery, the patient will require a period of controlled ventilation in the recovery room. Although many different types of mechanical ventilator are available, recovery staff must be familiar with the operation of the one in use in their unit.

The ventilator controls and gas flows are set by the anaesthetist but the recovery staff must know how to convert to manual ventilation should mechanical ventilation become unsatisfactory.

They may be required to monitor:

1. The respiratory rate.
2. The tidal volume (which can be read from a Wright spirometer placed on the expiratory limb of the ventilator tubing).
3. The minute volume (tidal volume × respiratory rate).
4. The airway pressure. This is the pressure required to inflate the lungs. It usually falls to zero during expiration unless positive and expiratory pressure (PEEP) is added.
5. The percentage of oxygen being delivered (an oxygen meter may be inserted into the gas supply).

Regardless of the type of ventilator in use and the settings on the dials, the chest must be seen to be expanding during inspiration and the patient's colour maintained. The ventilator may become disconnected or accidentally switched off and a ventilator alarm is advisable to alert nursing staff if this happens.

The anaesthetist must be informed immediately if:

1. The patient's colour deteriorates or the oxygen saturation reading on the oximeter falls.
2. The patient begins to resist the ventilator.
3. The airway pressures alter.
4. There are major fluctuations in the pulse or blood pressure.

OXYGEN THERAPY

The supply of oxygen to the tissues depends on three factors:

1. The delivery of oxygen to the blood stream by the respiratory system.
2. The uptake of oxygen by adequate amounts of normal haemoglobin.
3. The transport of oxygenated haemoglobin to the tissues by the cardiovascular system.

Even young fit patients who have received a brief anaesthetic may benefit from oxygen therapy in the recovery period since all general anaesthetics can depress respiration. In addition, if nitrous oxide has been used, it dilutes the oxygen in the alveoli as it comes out of solution in the first few minutes after its administration (Fink effect). Following prolonged anaesthesia, a period of 30-minutes' oxygen therapy will usually be sufficient to reduce hypoxaemia while the major depressant effects of anaesthesia are being eliminated (Meikeljohn, 1987).

Additional indications for oxygen therapy in the post-anaesthetic period include:

1. *Any abnormality of respiration:*
   - Poor respiratory effort
   - Lung disease (in the case of chronic bronchitis, see page 148)
   - Reduced diaphragmatic movement following high abdominal incision and in the obese
2. *Reduced or abnormal haemoglobin:*
   - Iron deficiency anaemia
   - Following severe haemorrhage
   - Sickle cell disease
3. *Abnormal cardiovascular system:*
   - Cardiac failure
   - Myocardial ischaemia
   - Cardiac irregularities
4. *When oxygen requirements are increased:*
   - Shivering
   - Thyrotoxicosis
   - Hyperpyrexia
5. *Restlessness and confusion:*
   - May signify cerebral hypoxia
6. *Whenever oxygen saturation is reduced or cyanosis is observed.*

ADMINISTRATION OF OXYGEN

Oxygen may come from a central piped supply or from cylinders. In the latter case, spares must always be available. Ball and tube flowmeters are generally used, the base of the ball giving the correct reading. Where rotameters are used, readings are taken from the top of the bobbin, which must be seen to be rotating.

Oxygen masks should cover the nose and mouth, be well fitting and made of a clear plastic or vinyl material so that the colour of the lips can be reviewed. Although many different methods are available for oxygen delivery, two are commonly used in recovery units:

1. *Simple plastic moulded face masks, e.g. Hudson Mask or MC Mask* (Figure 2.11). These are variable performance types of mask, the inspired oxygen concentration (F_iO_2) varying with the flow rate and the patient's minute volume. At flows of 6 l/min an inspired oxygen concentration of approximately 60% can generally be achieved, but this varies with the type of mask, and the manufacturer's instructions should be followed. At low flow rates rebreathing may occur.

2. *Venturi masks.* A supply of oxygen enriches entrained air by the Venturi principle, known as high air-flow oxygen enrichment (HAFOE) (Figure 2.12, *overleaf*). The oxygen port is graduated to give a range of F_iO_2 between 24% and 36%. This type of mask is used when controlled oxygen concentrations are required, e.g. in patients with chronic bronchitis (see page 148).

Patients should be told why they have a face mask in place in case they assume that they are still being anaesthetised. If a face mask is not tolerated, the use of nasal cannulae can provide a suitable alternative.

For the patient who is intubated, has a laryngeal mask airway or a tracheostomy, oxygen can be supplied via a T-piece system, the expiratory limb preventing dilution with air (Figure 2.13, *overleaf*). For the longer-stay patient, the gases should be warmed and humidified.

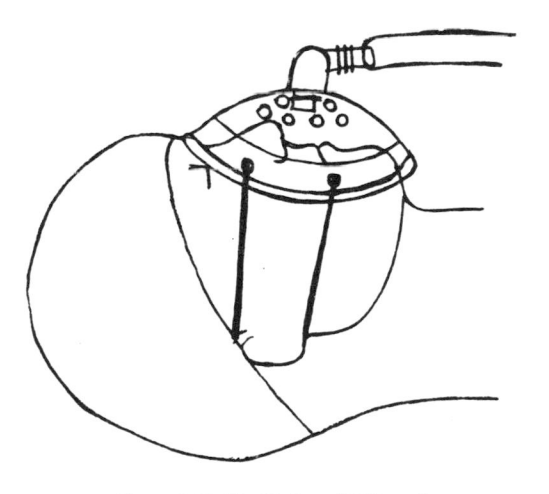

Figure 2.11 The Hudson (MC) mask

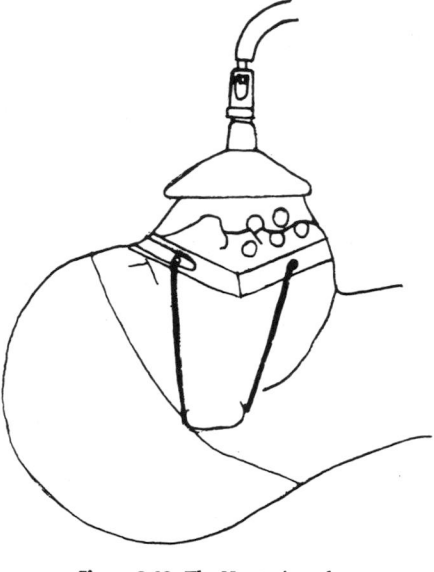

Figure 2.12 The Venturi mask

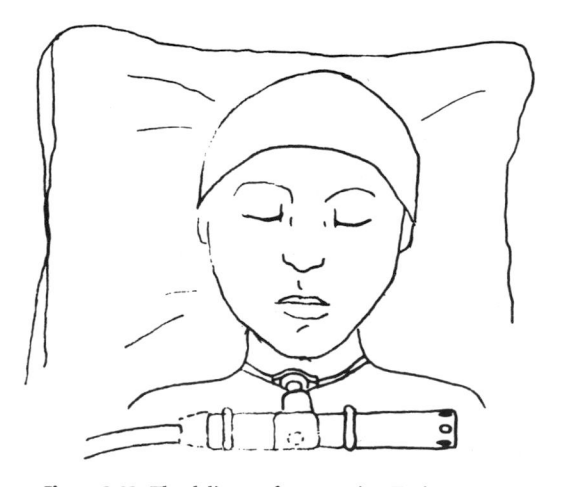

Figure 2.13 The delivery of oxygen via a T-piece system

If 100% oxygen is required, this can be provided using a closely fitting anaesthetic face mask and a Mapleson C circuit (Figure 2.14). With spontaneous breathing, the Heidbrink valve is fully open to minimise expiratory resistance. With controlled ventilation the valve is partially closed to allow pressure to be generated in the reservoir bag for inflation of the lungs.

Heidbrink valve

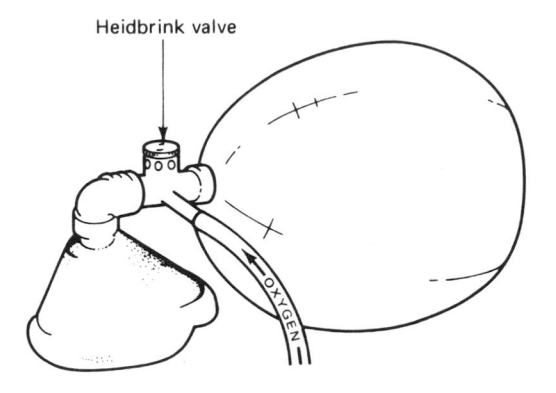

Figure 2.14 Mapleson C circuit with face mask

MAINTENANCE OF FLUID BALANCE

Measurement of post-operative fluid balance is vitally important. Assessment of fluid balance over a 12- or 24-hour period will frequently commence in the recovery period, so that it is essential that accurate records of both input and output, including all drainage systems, are assessed from the time of admission.

During those operative procedures requiring intravenous fluid therapy many factors will have been taken into account when deciding on the replacement regime. These include:

1. The pre-operative condition of the patient, e.g. state of hydration, electrolyte results, haemoglobin concentration, cardiac function.
2. The fasting period pre-operatively.
3. The patient's temperature and the ambient temperatures.
4. Evaporation from exposed tissues during surgery.
5. Blood loss during surgery and anticipated blood loss post-operatively.
6. Renal function.

Although the intravenous regimen may have been prescribed to cover the anticipated requirements of the subsequent 24 hours, it may require review during the immediate post-operative period as dictated by changes in the patient's clinical condition. Recovery-unit staff should refer at once to the anaesthetist for advice when such changes occur.

If signs of hypovolaemia develop, the infusion rate is increased and evidence of haemorrhage sought. The signs of hypovolaemia include:

1. Pallor.
2. Weak thready pulse.
3. Cold extremities.
4. Collapsed veins.
5. Increasing heart rate.

6. Falling blood pressure (this may be a late sign owing to compensatory vaso-constriction).
7. Oliguria.
8. Thirst.

Signs of circulatory overload must also be recognised as a dangerous situation which can be compounded unless fluids are restricted in patients with poor cardiac reserve. Such signs include:

1. Distended veins.
2. Full bounding pulse.
3. Increasing blood pressure.
4. Tachycardia.
5. Breathlessness.

INTRAVENOUS FLUID THERAPY

The integrity of the body will always have been violated by venepuncture and venous cannulation. Due precautions must therefore be taken to maintain sterility before, during and at the completion of intravenous therapy.
This will include the use of:

1. Sterile techniques.
2. Sterile apparatus.
3. Sterile fluids.
4. Sterile dressing.

INTRAVENOUS INFUSIONS

Personnel should first wash their hands and, though a sterile trolley is seldom required for setting up an intravenous infusion (IVI), the sterility of the equipment must be maintained by assuring that no connecting parts become contaminated at assembly. The wearing of gloves is advisable, not only in the interests of sterility, but also to give protection in case of accidental blood spillage. The site of the IVI should be cleansed with a spirit-based skin preparation and shaved if necessary. The optimal size of cannula varies according to the size of the vein selected and the type of fluid to be transfused. As the rate of infusion is directly proportional to the fourth power of the radius and inversely proportional to the viscosity of the fluid, a large cannula, e.g. 14G, is advisable if blood or packed cells are to be transfused. A sterile occlusive dressing with a securing tape both to cover and to anchor the cannula should be used.

INTRAVENOUS INFUSION DRIP RATES

Table 2.4 indicates the drip rate required to infuse 500 ml of fluid in a given time using a standard giving set from which 1 ml of fluid is normally delivered by approximately 16–18 drops. (Using the Metriset with paediatric patients the calculation is simpler as 60 drops = 1 ml. Therefore the number of drops per minute is the same as the number of millilitres per hour.)

Table 2.4. Intravenous infusion drip rates

Duration of infusion (h)	Drip rate drops/minute (approx.)
8	18
6	24
4	36
3	48
2	72
1	144

If the rate of an infusion is to be controlled mechanically by a syringe driver or pump then the required rate must be recorded on the prescription sheet and the concentration clearly marked on the side of the container or syringe.

INTRAVENOUS INJECTIONS

These should preferably be given by medical staff, but qualified nursing staff who have received the appropriate training and have the necessary authorisation may administer drugs intravenously through previously placed cannulae. Most hospitals have developed their own guidelines to cover:

1. The different methods by which nurses may give drugs intravenously.
2. The procedures to be followed in giving and recording drugs by each method.
3. Those authorised to give drugs by each method.
4. The rate at which each drug should be administered.
5. The amount and type of fluid which should be used if a drug needs to be diluted.
6. The type and amount of a drug that a nurse may give.

BLOOD TRANSFUSION

To increase the rate of infusion, a bag of blood can be compressed using a simple pressure bag, or, in cases of extreme urgency, a more sophisticated device such as the Kimal Rapid Infuser (Figure 2.15, *overleaf*).

A blood transfusion may already be in progress when the patient is admitted to the recovery unit in which case the checking procedures will already have been completed by the anaesthetist. However, if a transfusion of blood or blood products is due to begin while the patient is under the supervision of the recovery staff then the checking procedures must be strictly observed to ensure that the correct blood is given as clerical errors and inadequate checking are responsible for the majority of incompatible transfusions. The vital checking procedure is as follows:

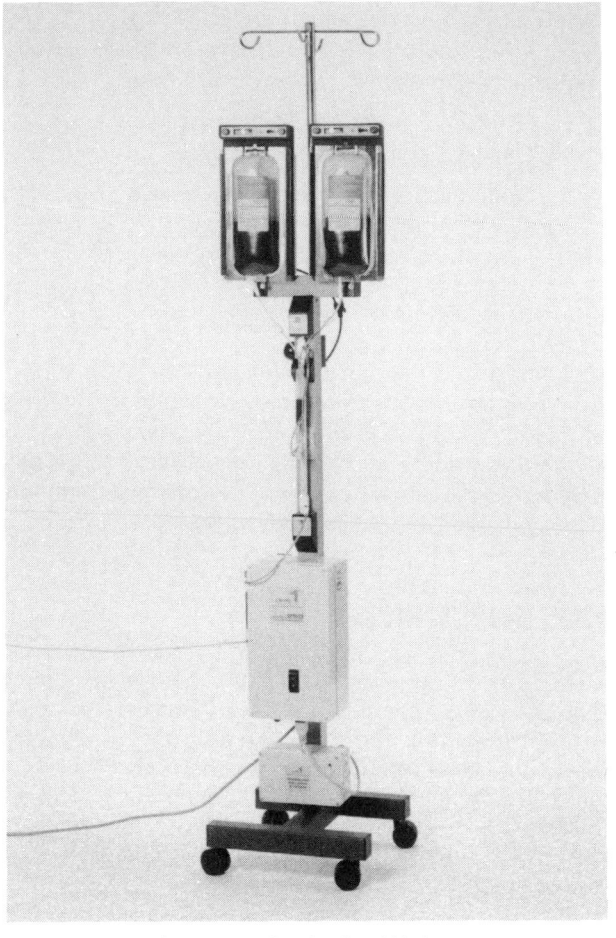

Figure 2.15 The Kimal rapid infuser

1. The patient's full name and hospital registration number must correspond to those on the blood unit label.
2. The blood group and Rhesus factor on the cross-match form must correspond to the blood unit label. In the case of rare groups, special arrangements are occasionally made with the transfusion laboratory for the supply of compatible blood of a different group. It is acceptable to infuse Rhesus positive into a Rhesus negative male but Rhesus positive blood should *never* be given to a Rhesus negative woman of child-bearing potential.
3. The blood unit number must correspond with the patient's blood-transfusion form.
4. The expiry date must not have passed. Checking must be assiduous and no discrepancy either in the spelling of the patient's name or in the legibility of letters or numbers should be accepted. Once the blood has been checked

and confirmed as satisfactory, the transfusion form is signed beside the corresponding unit number, witnessed by an assistant, and the transfusion commenced. The time is noted.

The patient must be observed frequently at the commencement of each transfusion so that reactions can be identified without delay (see page 103).

Blood should remain refrigerated until it is required. It should not be removed for more that 30 min before administration, in order to avoid the risk of multiplication of any previous bacterial contamination.

When large volumes are given rapidly, closer observation is required as additional hazards may be encountered (pages 104–109), and the blood units should be warmed as transfused.

Special consideration is required in the management of Jehovah's Witnesses. Their religion forbids the transfusion of blood and blood products and their wishes must be respected. In the case of an emergency admission where no history is available and where the patient is unconscious in the recovery room, every effort must be made to discover their religious beliefs before commencing a transfusion. Most hospitals have an agreed policy for the guidance of staff.

DRAINAGE SYSTEMS

When recording fluid balance, all drainage systems should be included, the amount and character or colour of the fluid being described. The following are used in the recovery unit:

1. *Urine drainage* (see page 109).
2. *Nasogastric tube drainage.* When a nasogastric tube is *in situ*, it should be aspirated early in an attempt to empty the stomach. Although this cannot be assured using a narrow gauge tube, it will, however, reduce intragastric pressure and make regurgitation less likely. It should then be left on open drainage with the drainage bag secured at a level lower than the patient's stomach. The tube should be secured at the nose and again over the forehead or at the temple. The integrity of the cardiac sphincter has been breached by the presence of the tube which, if blocked or kinked, will not prevent vomiting or regurgitation taking place around the tube. If the patient appears nauseated, suction should at once be applied to the tube. A record of the amount and nature of the fluid obtained should be made. It is preferable for the nasogastric tube to be introduced while the patient is anaesthetised as attempts to do so during the recovery phase are unpleasant for the patient and may promote vomiting.
3. *T-tube drainage.* A T-tube is inserted at surgery when the common bile duct has been explored – choledochostomy. It provides a safety valve when oedema may obstruct the flow of bile through the sphincter of Oddi with a consequent possible leakage into the peritoneum. It is required, therefore, as an overflow, not for the total drainage of the bile. Large quantities of bile

would only be seen if a complete obstruction existed in the common bile duct and would even then not be seen until later when the patient was returned to the ward. It is preferable *not* to secure the bag with a safety pin, but with adhesive plaster. In restless patients the tube could be pulled from the wound (Allan, 1977). It is important that the bag is level with the patient and not beneath the bed or trolley in case a syphon effect should be created.

4. *Ileostomy and colostomy bags.* These need to be directed towards the feet and not across the patient, because when he is sitting upright, there will be a gravitational flow. An emission of faecal fluid is unlikely in the immediate recovery period but the stoma area should be observed for blood loss. The adhesive fit between the neck of the collecting apparatus and the skin must be maintained.

5. *Vacuum drainage bottles.* When the antennae on top of the bottle are pointing laterally the bottle is at a negative pressure and functioning correctly. If there is a loss of vacuum, i.e. with the antennae vertical, further suction can be applied to the bottle. A sterile rigid sucker end should be used. Further vacuum failure will require the advice of the surgeon. If no fluid drains along the tubing to the bottle, an inspection must be made at the site of entry to the tissues for evidence of swelling or haematoma. This might indicate that the proximal end of the tube is blocked. The surgeon should then be consulted.

6. *Bellow drains – low vacuum.* The compressible plastic containers must be checked for maintenance of vacuum. They are used for superficial tissue drainage. As there can be no graduated marks on this type of apparatus, the volumes they contain cannot be accurately measured but the amounts are usually small.

7. *Chest drainage* (see page 131).

8. *Bladder irrigation* (see page 135).

RECORD KEEPING AND CHARTING

For the understanding of the needs of any one patient, and to promote a skilled and intelligent approach to recovery nursing, the recovery unit will require a charting system designed for its special needs. One of its main functions, other than being an accurate record, is its use as a tool. Serial recordings will show improving or stable parameters or swiftly reveal trends which require immediate correction. An interpretation must be made and an understanding of the physiological signs is required. Anything less than this is to ignore the importance of this short-term vital charting. The chart should be of adequate size and have an identifiable colour. At the top of the chart there should be space for:

1. Patient identification.

2. Relevant medical history.

3. Drug history.
4. Relevant pre-operative recordings, e.g. weight, blood pressure, heart rate and haemoglobin concentration.

There should be space on the chart to record:

1. Time of observation.
2. Colour and oxygen saturation.
3. Respiratory rate and depth.
4. Pulse rate and rhythm.
5. Blood pressure.
6. Level of consciousness.
7. Temperature.
8. Oxygen concentration administration.
9. Intravenous infusion.
10. Drug therapy.
11. Operation site review.
12. Recovery nurse's signature.

A simple example is given in Figure 2.16 (*overleaf*). The reverse side is available for continuation.

The information above the double line is completed pre-operatively in the anaesthetic room or reception area by the recovery staff and the chart is then sent to the recovery unit. It is then attached to a clipboard at the patient's bay to await his admission. The example shown allows for observations over a period of 1 h 40 min. As the average length of a patient's stay is 30–45 min, it covers a satisfactory time span in most cases.

A continuation of the anaesthetic record chart is used by some recovery units, marking their observations in red at the changeover. They are, however, ill-suited for recording the special observations necessary for the recovery service. This also applies to the design of the surgical ward chart. On the other hand, when a specific recovery room chart is used, the ward staff can easily continue to record their observations on it, as it has all the features needed to review the patient's immediate post-operative state. The clinical signs are clear to read in sequence, any one line of observations showing an easy evaluation which relates to previous recordings.

If a patient requires ventilatory support in his recovery time, a special chart should be provided (Figure 2.17, *overleaf*).

The accurate recording of the patient's progress after a given anaesthetic is of great value should further surgery be required. It may also be of great import for medico-legal cases when the recovery charting and the staff carrying out patient care will come under close scrutiny.

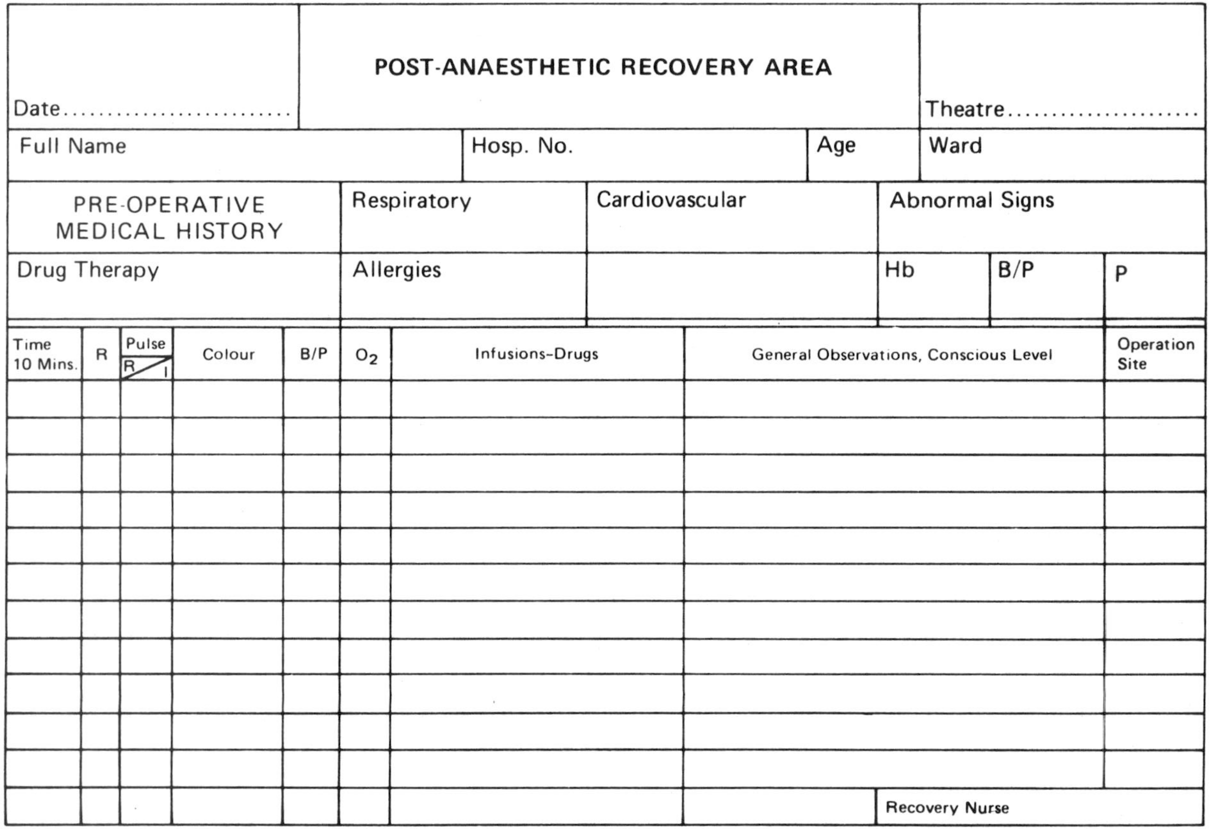

POST-ANAESTHETIC RECOVERY AREA

Date................

Full Name................ Hosp. No. Age Ward Theatre....................

PRE-OPERATIVE MEDICAL HISTORY	Respiratory	Cardiovascular	Abnormal Signs		
Drug Therapy	Allergies		Hb	B/P	P

Time 10 Mins.	Pulse R / R / I	Colour	B/P	O₂	Infusions–Drugs	General Observations, Conscious Level	Operation Site
					Recovery Nurse		

Figure 2.16 Recovery room chart

Recovery Observation Chart — Ventilator Care

DATE	NAME	AGE	REG No	WARD	VENTILATOR	ENDOTRACHEAL / TRACHEOSTOMY TUBE SIZE - CUFF INFLATION: m/s

TIME	RESP/MIN	MIN VOL	TIDAL VOL	Pressure CM	O₂ /Lt	AIR /Lt	N₂O /Lt	PULSE	B/p	TEMP	CVP	Suction	Turning	OP: Site Check	DRUGS - Dose - Route Frequency

TIME	INVESTIGATIONS	Blood Gases	Hb	Urea - Electrolytes	BLOOD SUGAR	CHEST X-RAY	ECG	PROTHROBIN TIME	DOCTOR'S SIGNATURE

NURSE'S SIGNATURE - - - - - - - - - - -

Figure 2.17 Recovery room chart for ventilated patients

CRITERIA FOR DISCHARGE

Discharge to a Ward

Before each patient is discharged to a ward, the recovery staff must be satisfied that:

- The patient is fully conscious, his reflexes have returned and he can protect his airway.
- Breathing is adequate, a good central colour is maintained and the oxygen saturation is satisfactory.
- The cardiovascular system is stable. Consecutive readings of pulse and blood pressure approximate to normal pre-operative values, peripheral perfusion is good and there is no unexplained cardiac irregularity and no persistent bleeding.
- The patient is comfortable, and not in pain. Patients should remain in the recovery unit for 30 min following the administration of drugs such as respiratory stimulants or vasopressers to enable their effects to be observed. The anaesthetist should re-examine the patient to ensure that repeat administration is not required. The assessment of blood transfusions also may delay a patient's return to the ward.
- Nerve blocks have receded. The patient is able to appreciate light touch and motor function has returned (page 57).

Once the above criteria have been met, the patient and the linen are clean and the paperwork is complete, it is then safe to return the patient to the ward. Before contact with the ward is made, the discharge must first be sanctioned by the anaesthetist or by a deputy nominated by him.

Under no circumstances should a patient be discharged prematurely from a recovery area into the care of possibly less-experienced staff on a ward. In the dimmed lighting of a ward at night, this may become an added problem. In hospitals with an emergency surgical service, recovery facilities must be available at all times (i.e. throughout the 24 hours and at weekends). In those hospitals that undertake little emergency surgery, the anaesthetist and operating staff should monitor the patient's recovery until it is safe for him to return to his ward.

Failure to provide adequate nursing care for patients during a period in which they are vulnerable and at risk of serious complications is unacceptable. Not only is the patient's life and well-being endangered, but it may also prove extremely expensive for those responsible.

Once all the above criteria have been met and the patient's discharge has been approved by the anaesthetist or his deputy, the ward should be contacted to ensure that they are ready to take over care. The patient should be accompanied by a trained and experienced nurse and porter.

In the case of day surgery, additional criteria are required before the patient can return home (page 167).

Discharge to Intensive Care or High-dependency Unit

Should a patient's recovery from anaesthesia be prolonged or complicated, it may become necessary for him to be transferred to an intensive care or high-dependency unit rather than to return to a general surgical ward. It is obviously an advantage if these units are close to the main recovery area since transfer over a large distance can be hazardous. All patients should be adequately monitored during transfer. If transfer to a specialised unit is delayed, the recovery unit should be able to provide short-term intensive care including mechanical ventilation.

TRANSFER OF PATIENT TO WARD STAFF

A trained member of the ward nursing staff or recovery room should escort the patient from the recovery unit. They should be given the following information (but not within the hearing of the patient):

1. The patient's name.
2. The nature of the surgery performed.
3. The names of the surgeon and the anaesthetist.
4. The anaesthetic technique used, e.g. general, regional, hypotensive.
5. The relevant information concerning drains, catheters, packs and suture materials.
6. The progress of the patient in the recovery period.
7. The post-operative requirements concerning oxygen therapy, position and frequency of observations.

The anaesthetic record, the recovery room chart and the prescription sheet all accompany the patient to the ward.

If recovery-room equipment accompanies a patient to the ward a record should be made to this effect in order to ensure its return when no longer required.

References and Bibliography

Association of Anaesthetists of Great Britain and Ireland (AAGBI) (1991). The High Dependency Unit.

Allan D (1977). Complications of T tube drainage. Nursing Times, Aug, 1270–1271.

Allen D (1988). Making sense of suction. Nursing Times, 84(10), 46–47.

American Medical Association (1988). General principles of blood transfusions. AMA, Monro, Wisconsin, USA.

Andrewes SJ (1979). The recovery room as a nursing service. J R Soc Med, 72, 275–277.

Bambridge AD (1993). Nasal catheters for oxygen administration: an audit of safety and patient comfort. Br J Theat Nurs, Jan, 2(10).

Canadian Association of Critical Care Nurses (1992). Standards for critical care nursing practice, 50, London, Ontario, Canada, 28.

Craig DB (1981). Post-operative recovery of pulmonary function. Anaes Analg, 60, 46–52.

Dale RF, Lindop MJ, Farman JV, Smith MF (1986). Autotransfusions, an experience of 76 cases. Annals Roy Col Surg, 68, 295–297.

Dexter F, Tinker JH (1995). Analysis of strategies to decrease post-anaesthesia care unit costs. Anesthesiol, 82(1), Jan., 94–101.

Drain CB, Shipley SB (1997). The recovery room. A critical care approach to post-anaesthetic nursing. WB Saunders Company, Philadelphia.

Guedel AE (1933). JAMA, 100, 1862. Reprinted in 'Classical File', Surv Anaesthesiol, 10, 515 (1966).

Hatfield A, Tronson M (1994). The Complete Recovery Room Book, OUP.

Johnson B (1993). The ABC's of recovery room nursing. Can Op Room Nurs J, 11(2), May–Jun, 6–11.

Kember NF (1982). An introduction to computer application in medicine. Edward Arnold, London.

Kinney JM, Bendixen HH, Powers SR (1977). Manual of surgical intensive care. WB Saunders, Philadelphia/London.

Kirkendall MD, Burton AC, Epstein FM, Freis ED (1967). Recommendations for human blood pressure determinations by sphygmomanometers. American Heart Association.

Kurth CD (1995). Post-operative arterial oxygen saturation: what to expect (editorial). Anesth Analg, 80(1), Jan, 1-3.

Levine A, Imai P (1983). Autotransfusions. Am Op Room Nurses, 37(6), USA, 1061–1064.

Lunn JN (1994). Recovery from anaesthesia. BMJ, 308(6932), 804.

Lyon MH, West BJM (1994). Immediate post-operative recovery: measurement and care. Br J Nurs, 3(17), Sep 22-Oct 12, 866, 868–870.

Meikeljohn BH (1987). Arterial oxygen desaturation during post-operative transportation. Anaes, 42, 1313–1315.

Milne C (1988). Computers in nursing. Nursing Stand, 2(37), 32–33.

Nicholson E (1988). Autologous blood transfusions. Nursing Times, 84(2), 33–35.

Pearsall FJ, Davidson JA, Asbury AJ (1995). The attitudes to the Association of Anaesthetists recommendations for standards of monitoring during anaesthesia and recovery. Anaesthes, 50(7), Jul, 649–653.

Pollock AV, Evans M (1991). Post-operative complications in surgery. Blackwell Scientific, Oxford.

Prowse M (1995). Toward 2001. The recovery room revisited. Br J Theat Nurs, 4(12), March, 6–7.

Wallace CJ (1981). Anaesthetic nursing. Pitman Medical, London.

Ward CS (1985). Anaesthetic equipment, 2nd edn. Baillière Tindall, London.

Wilson R, Gaer J (1988). Right atrial electrocardiography in placement of central venous catheters. Lancet, 1, 462–463.

Chapter 3
PAIN RELIEF AND LOCAL ANAESTHESIA

INTRODUCTION

Surgery is almost invariably associated with pain and very few patients do not require post-operative analgesia. It is difficult to provide consistently effective post operative pain relief while avoiding side-effects. Although standards are rapidly rising, the failure to provide comprehensive post-operative pain relief to all patients has been rightly criticised as one of modern medicine's greatest failings.

GATE-CONTROL THEORY OF PAIN

It is now over 30 years since Melzack and Wall (1965, 1989) proposed their theory of the gate-control of pain (Figure 3.1, *overleaf*). They postulate that painful stumuli are transmitted by a variety of nerve fibres with differing conduction rates to cells in the dorsal horn of the spinal column. These cells may either allow the stimuli to pass on to the brain, where they are perceived as pain, or terminated within the cord. These cells act as a gate – if it is "open" pain is felt; if it is "closed" it is not. The gate may be closed by other peripheral nerve fibres or by descending central inhibitory fibres. Peripheral inhibition can be initiated by friction (rubbing it better), counter-irritants, muscle activity or transcutaneous nerve stimulation (TENS). An example of central inhibition (mind over matter) would be the sportsman who does not notice an injury until the game is over.

An ever increasing number of neuro-transmitter substances are being identified that play a role in either the perception of pain or its inhibition. Much interest has centred on the endorphins – short-acting morphine-like substances synthesised by the body. As they are found in the cerebrospinal fluid, synthetic opiates are now frequently injected into the intrathecal or epidural spaces in attempts to mirror and improve on their action.

Although most patients expect to experience some discomfort after surgery, no one should be allowed to remain in pain in the PACU nor be discharged back to their ward without their pain being relieved. The amount of pain experienced by a given patient will vary and each patient must be assessed individually. It follows that their analgesic requirements will also vary and that there is no such thing as a routine dose of painkiller.

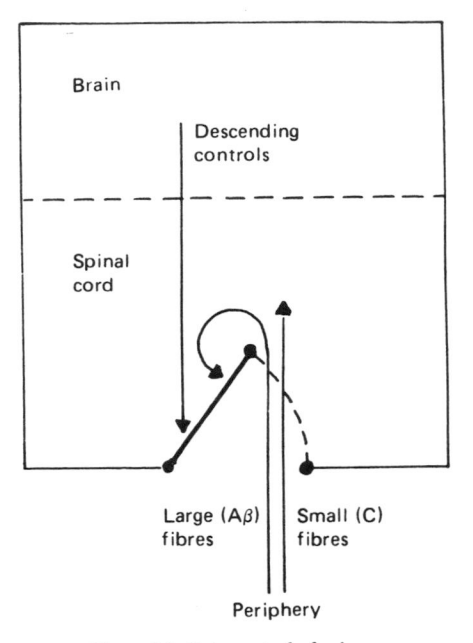

Figure 3.1 Gate control of pain

Factors that influence the amount of pain experienced post-operatively include:

1. The site of the operation.
2. Analgesics given pre- or intra-operatively.
3. The concomitant use of a local anaesthetic blockade.
4. The patient's personality and state of mind.

Patients who say that they are in pain should be believed even if their operation was "minor" and not usually associated with a great deal of post-operative discomfort. Particular attention should be paid to patients who cannot easily communicate their distress. These include:

1. Infants and young children.
2. Patients who are intubated or have a tracheostomy.
3. The mentally handicapped.
4. Patients whose native language is not English.

Signs of inadequate pain relief may include:

1. Restlessness.
2. Hypertension.
3. Tachycardia.
4. Sweating or lachrymation.
5. Rapid shallow respiration.

METHODS OF PAIN RELIEF

Analgesic Drugs

Narcotic Analgesics

Opiates remain the drugs most commonly used for post-operative analgesia. Prescribers often have a preferred opiate but there is probably little to choose between them when they are used for acute pain relief. All the commonly used drugs (morphine, pethidine, fentanyl, etc) are equally effective providing adequate amounts are given at appropriate time intervals. All have the same potential side-effects:

1. Respiratory depression.
2. Nausea and vomiting.
3. Hypotension.
4. Sedation.
5. Pupillary constriction.
6. Smooth muscle contraction leading to possible bronchoconstriction, biliary or renal colic and constipation.

The first three listed are the most important in the PACU, and if encountered should be treated immediately.

Should serious respiratory depression occur, it can be readily reversed with intravenous naloxone. Unless, however, the dose of naloxone is carefully titrated against the patient's respiratory depression, it will also reverse analgesia. For this reason, many prefer to treat depressed respiration with incremental intravenous doxapram, which will stimulate respiration without reversing analgesia. It should also be remembered that naloxone is a short-acting agent. It is therefore possible for patients to suffer a second period of respiratory depression after apparent recovery, especially if they have been given an intramuscular or subcutaneous bolus of opiate.

Nausea and vomiting are common side-effects of opiates especially after middle-ear surgery and some gynaecological operations, but they are not inevitable. Anti-emetics are probably best not given routinely as they produce sideeffects of their own. It is, nevertheless, wise to ensure that they have been prescribed so that they can be given if indicated.

Although many opiates can be given orally, rectally and now buccally and transcutaneously, as well as by injection, the intravenous route is to be preferred when rapid relief is required. Small increments of the chosen drug should be given and their effect monitored as there is no "routine" or maximum dose. The correct dose is that which relieves the patient's pain. If an unusually large dose seems to be required, it is wise to examine the injection site to confirm that the cannula is in the vein. Other simple, treatable causes of pain, such as a full bladder, should be excluded. Very anxious or nervous patients may complain of pain but will respond to explanation and reassurance.

The intramuscular route, although widely used, is very much a second best option. Absorption from the injection site is slow and adequate analgesia may not be obtained for 30 min or more, especially if tissue perfusion is impaired by hypotension or peripheral vasoconstriction. Furthermore, titration to optimal analgesia is very difficult with alternating poor analgesia or over sedation.

Occasionally, the oral or rectal routes may be sensible options, but allowance must always be made for the slower rate of absorption. Recently, attention has focused on the use of the subcutaneous route, especially in infants and children. A butterfly-type needle or cannula is placed subcutaneously and incremental doses of narcotic are given until adequate analgesia is obtained. This method is said to be much less painful than repeated intramuscular injections.

Particular care should be exercised when opiates are administered to:

1. Patients with chronic respiratory disease.
2. Patients who have undergone neurosurgery or had a recent head injury.
3. Patients taking monoamine oxidase inhibitors.
4. Children and elderly patients.
5. Hypotensive patients.

The judicious use of opiates may allow a patient with chronic respiratory disease to breathe more easily and co-operate with their physiotherapists, while adequate analgesia may allow a head-injury patient to be more adequately assessed. It is a myth that infants and the elderly feel less pain than other age groups – they should be given analgesia like all other patients, but the optimal dose needs to be assessed carefully as they may be more sensitive to the drugs' side-effects and require relatively smaller doses. If possible, non-opiate analgesics or regional anaesthetic techniques should be considered.

It is also a myth that addiction can result from appropriate post-operative prescribing. The short-term use of narcotics for post-operative analgesia almost never leads to habituation. Adequate analgesia should be provided without worrying about rare hypothetical dangers.

Oral preparations of most opiates and rectal preparations of a few are available and are potentially useful for post-operative analgesia. Oral morphine has an onset time of 20–30 min and lasts for approximately 4 h. Long-acting opiate preparations of morphine (e.g. MST) or fentanyl (durogesic) are neither suitable nor licensed for post-operative use and should not be used.

Partial Antagonists

Buprenorphine, meptazinol, nalbuphine and pentazocine differ from other potent analgesics in that they have both agonist and antagonist properties, i.e. they both bind to opiate receptors and also block the action of other opiates at them. They can, theoretically, reverse the actions of opiate agonists and precipitate withdrawal reactions. They are effective analgesics and until recently were not subject to Schedule 2 of the Misuse of Drugs Regulations (UK) so that no register had to be completed before they were administered. Buprenorphine and pentazocine are, however, now controlled drugs. They often show a "ceiling effect", i.e. above a given dose, no better analgesia results but side-effects may be greater. Their side-effect profile is similar to other opiates but with, perhaps, less respiratory depression but a higher incidence of dysphoria and hallucinations. As the sequential use of opiate agonists and partial antagonists can lead to a pharmacological muddle, their use in the PACU is, probably, best avoided.

Patient-controlled Analgesia

A recent innovation that has rapidly gained wide-spread popularity has been the development of patient-controlled analgesia (PCA). A syringe of analgesic is connected to a dedicated intravenous cannula, i.e. the cannula is not used for other purposes. The syringe is attached to a programmable electronic pump with a hand-set for the patient to use. When the button on the hand-set is pressed, a predetermined bolus of analgesic is delivered intravenously. The pump is programmed with the drug concentration, the size of bolus to be delivered, the lock-out time between boluses and the rate of background infusion to be administered. Many pumps can also be interrogated to determine the amount of analgesic that the patient has self-administered.

Patients who have used PCAs generally express a high level of satisfaction with the quality of their post-operative analgesia even if they have self-administered lower doses of analgesics than comparable patients receiving conventional intramuscular injections. It is noteworthy that apparently similar patients undergoing identical surgery self-administer widely differing amounts of analgesic but with comparable levels of satisfaction, emphasising yet again, how variable are patients' post-operative analgesic requirements.

Patients undergoing major surgery who will be offered a post-operative PCA should be shown the equipment pre-operatively and have its use explained to them. This task often falls to the PACU staff who work as part of an acute pain-management team. In our hospital, morphine is our drug of choice and is prepared as a 1 mg/ml solution. 2.5–5 mg of droperidol is generally added to each 50 mg of morphine to reduce the incidence of post-operative nausea and vomiting. Bolus doses of 1–1.5 mg of morphine are delivered with a 5 min lockout period. Background infusions are not used.

Suitable charts for prescribing patient-controlled analgesia and for monitoring patients receiving it are illustrated in Figures 3.2 and 3.3 (*overleaf*).

Balanced Analgesia

Recently the concept of balanced analgesia has become popular. Essentially, improved analgesia is sought through the use of several different techniques or analgesic drugs with different modes of action. Commonly, opiates are supplemented with non-steroidal anti-inflammatory drugs (NSAIDs) and local anaesthetic blocks.

Non-steroidal Anti-inflammatory Drugs (NSAIDs)

This large group of drugs has been available in tablet or capsule form for many years for the management of musculo-skeletal pain. The recent introduction of injectible preparations together with suppositories, creams and gels has markedly extended their range of uses. They are increasingly used pre-, intra- and post-operatively as analgesics. They are, however, not without their side-effects – they can cause gastric irritation or bleeding, fluid retention, reduced renal perfusion and can exacerbate asthma is some susceptible individuals.

NAME ....

ADDRESS ....

....

....

DATE OF BIRTH ....

HOSP. NUMBER ....

attach addressograph if available

OPERATION: ....

SPECIALTY:

ENT .... ORTHO .... TRAUMA ....

GEN SURG .... UROLOGY .... GYNAE ....

VASCULAR ...... PAEDS .... HAEMATOLOGY ....

OTHER ....

additional patient details:

ASA GRADE: 1   2   3   4   5

WEIGHT: ....kg

PCA INFUSION AS FOLLOWS:
(anaesthetist to complete)

OPIOID: ....mg

ANTIEMETIC: droperidol   ....mg

        made up to ....ml with Normal Saline

ANAESTHETIST's DETAILS:

SURNAME .... *signed* ....

                        date ....

WARD ....

PUMP ....

CONCURRENT ANALGESIA
(for database information)
N.S.A.I.D.s   ....
LOCAL
ANAESTHETIC   ....
   how used? ....
   ....

LOADING DOSE initial dose (mg) in recovery		CHANGES TO PRESCRIPTION				
		date:	date:	date:	date:	date:
BOLUS (mg)						
LOCK-OUT DURATION time after completion of a successful demand that patient is prevented from receiving further boluses						
CONCENTRATION (mg/ml)						
BACKGROUND INFUSION (not used at GRH)						
TOTAL SINCE RESET (mg) total given since last reset						
DOCTOR's SIGNATURE						

DATE STARTED   .... / .... / ....

TIME STARTED   .... : ....

DATE STOPPED   .... / .... / ....

TIME STOPPED   .... : ....

TOTAL USED (mg)   ....

REASON FOR DISCONTINUATION
NO LONGER NEEDED   VENFLON FELL OUT
VENFLON TISSUED
OTHER ....
Comments:...
....

URINARY RETENTION *(while using P.C.A.)*
catheter sited at operation   no catheter used
catheterised postop   in & out catheterisation

Figure 3.2 Patient-controlled analgesia prescription

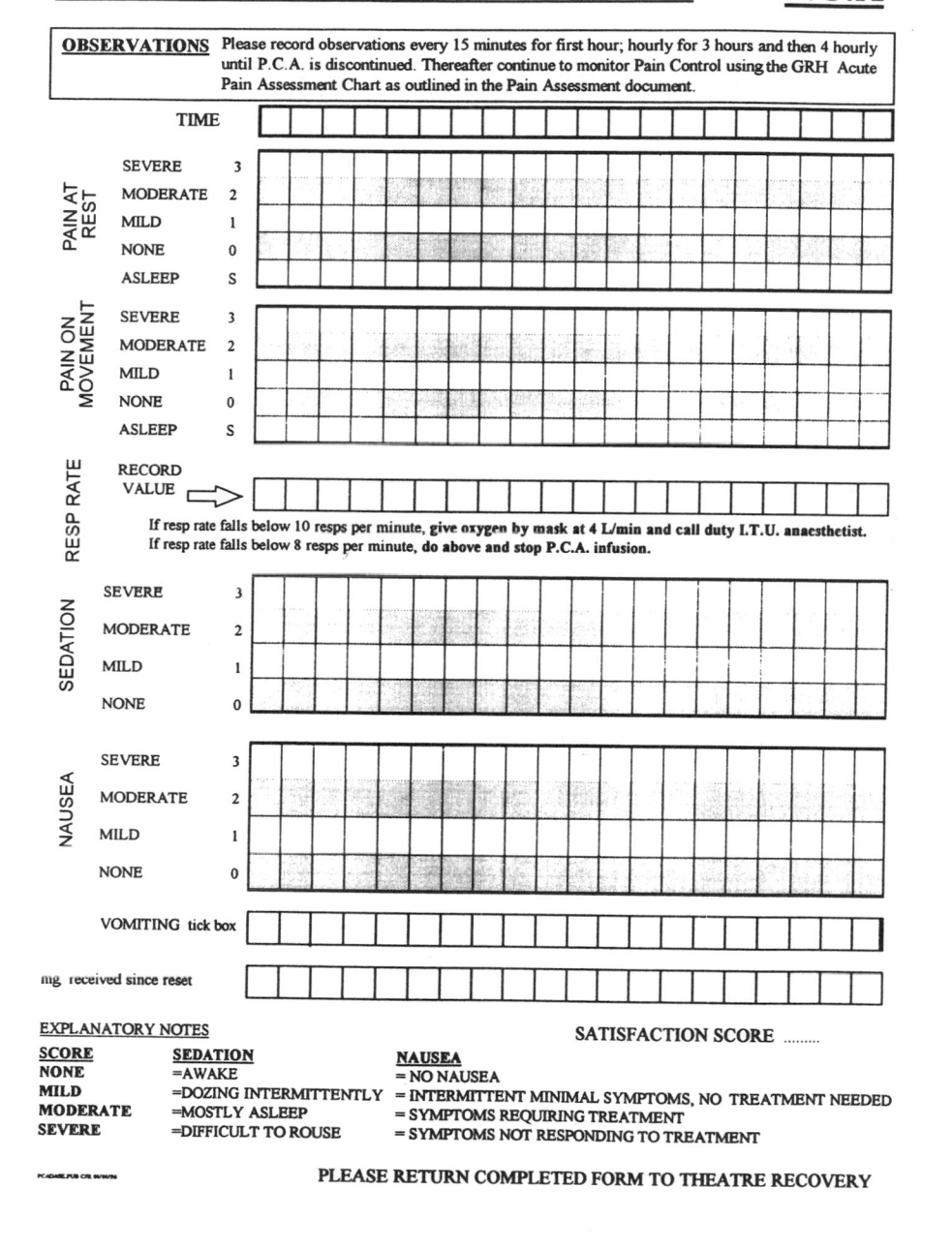

Figure 3.3 Patient-controlled analgesia observation record

Choosing an NSAID for Use in the Peri-operative Period

- NSAIDs are useful adjuncts for peri-operative analgesia and, because of their opioid-sparing effects, should be considered whenever opioids are used.
- They may be equipotent with opioids for some dental and orthopaedic procedures. They should not be used as the sole analgesic after major surgery.
- Exercise considerable caution with their use in patients with a history of gastro-duodenal bleeding, altered fluid balance and moderate/severe renal impairment.
- NSAIDs are contra-indicated in patients with a history of NSAID- or aspirin-induced bronchospasm. In other asthmatics, they may be used with caution.
- NSAIDs should be used with caution in patients on heparin or oral anti-coagulants.
- Intravenous NSAIDs are contra-indicated in patients on anticoagulants.
- The NSAID of choice is probably diclofenac as it combines efficacy with a reasonable safety profile. It is also available in standard, slow-release and soluble-oral formulations, as well as intravenous and intramuscular injectible preparations and suppositories.
- The oral route is to be preferred. Patients who are to be given a suppository after premedication or anaesthesia should be forewarned. Legal actions have occurred when anaesthetised patients have been given suppositories without their prior consent.

Paracetamol and Combination Analgesics

Paracetamol is a widely used simple analgesic that is useful for mild-to-moderate post-operative pain, either by itself or in combination with the weaker opiates (codeine, dihydrocodeine or dextropropoxyphene). It is a popular analgesic for young children as it is available as a suspension that can be given orally. Several preparations are available containing either 120 mg/5 ml or 250 mg/ 5ml. Recommended doses of the 120 mg/5 ml preparation are:

Under 3 months	2.5 ml	
3 months to 1 year	2.5–5 ml	} all four times a day.
1–6 years	5–10 ml	

Paracetamol suppositories (125 mg and 500 mg) are also available and may be used with good effect.

Adults undergoing minor surgery who can take oral analgesics are frequently prescribed combination analgesics post-operatively. An increasing number are available including:

Paracetamol 325 mg/dextropropoxyphene 32.5 mg	Co-proxamol
Paracetamol 500 mg/codeine 8 mg	Co-codamol
Paracetamol 500 mg/dihydrocodeine 10 mg	Co-dydramol

Paracetamol 500 mg/dihydrocodeine 20 mg	Remedeine
Paracetamol 500 mg/dihydrocodeine 30 mg	Remedeine Forte
Paracetamol 500 mg/codeine 30 mg	Tylex, Solpadol, Kapake

The maximum dose of all the preparations mentioned is 8 tablets/24 h. The first three preparations are generally well tolerated with few side-effects. The latter three are associated with a greater incidence of problems owing to the increased doses of opiate that they contain. If the maximum doses of these preparations are taken for more than a few days, constipation is likely to be a problem.

Local Anaesthetic Techniques

After a period during which they were little used, local anaesthetic blocks are regaining popularity both as an alternative and as an adjunct to general anaesthesia and for post-operative analgesia. Like every other technique, they have their advantages and disadvantages:

Advantages

- No loss of protective reflexes.
- Little cardiovascular or respiratory depression.
- Less systemic upset with negligible hang-over, little nausea or vomiting and a lower incidence of deep-vein thrombosis.
- Smooth pain-free recovery.

Disadvantages

- Time consuming to perform.
- Extra skill necessary to perform the block reliably.
- Co-operation from the patient and surgeon is necessary.
- They are useful for a restricted range of operations.
- They are contra-indicated in the presence of clotting defects or sepsis at the site of skin puncture.

Some of the problems and complications that can occur are common to all local anaesthetic procedures while others are specific to certain blocks. Complications may be either local, at or about the site of injection, or systemic.

Local Complications

These include:

- Infection.
- Ischaemia if adrenaline-containing solutions are used.
- Haematoma.
- Nerve damage.
- Damage to other local structures, e.g. pneumothorax.

Systemic Complications

These are due to either an excessively large dose of local anaesthetic being injected, an appropriate dose being too rapidly absorbed, or being injected inadvertently into a blood vessel or the cerebro-spinal fluid. They may be:

1. **Neurological:** restlessness, tremor, convulsions and medullary depression resulting in respiratory and cardiac depression. Total paralysis can follow the injection of an inappropriately large dose intrathecally.
2. **Cardiovascular:** tachycardia and hypertension (if adrenaline-containing solutions are used). Myocardial depression with bradycardia and hypotension if plain solutions are used.
3. **Psychogenic:** bradycardia and hypotension leading to fainting can be vagally mediated in nervous patients or those with a fear of needles.

Management of Toxic Reactions

As always, prevention is better than cure. The frequency of toxic reactions can be reduced by:

- Not exceeding the recommended dose of the local anaesthetic being used.
- Maintaining verbal contact with the patient while the block is being performed and during surgery.
- Aspirating frequently while injecting the local anaesthetic so as to detect rapidly inadvertent vessel puncture.
- Never using adrenaline-containing solutions in areas supplied by end arteries, e.g. fingers, toes and the penis.

Local anaesthetic blocks should never be performed if adequate resuscitation equipment is not immediately available.

Respiratory depression is treated with oxygen and artificial ventilation with a bag and mask, laryngeal mask airway or endotracheal intubation, as appropriate.

Cardiovascular depression is treated with oxygen, the rapid infusion of intravenous fluids, a head-down tilt, atropine and vasoconstrictors (e.g. ephedrine, phenylephrine or metaraminol).

Convulsions are treated with oxygen and intravenous diazepam.

Local Anaesthetic Agents

Only three local anaesthetic agents are currently available in the UK although a fourth (ropivacaine) is shortly to be launched. In other markets, a larger number is available. They are generally available as both plain solutions and with added adrenaline, or in the case of prilocaine, added felypressin. These agents are added to the local anaesthetic solution to produce local vasoconstriction which will slow absorption thus prolonging the duration of the block and reducing the risk of toxic side-effects.

When calculating doses of local anaesthetic, remember a 1% solution contains 10 mg/ml.

Lignocaine

This is the standard agent with which all others are compared. It is rapidly effective when injected and lasts for 60–90 min. A 1% solution will produce a sensory block of most nerves. More concentrated solutions (2%) are available if a motor block is required. A 4% solution can be used for topical anaesthesia of mucous membranes. The maximum recommended dose of the plain solution is of the order of 3 mg/kg, thus 200 mg can be given to an average adult and 400–500 mg if the adrenaline-containing solution is used.

Prilocaine

It is similar to lignocaine but has a greater therapeutic influence. Larger amounts may, therefore, be used: 300 mg of the plain solution and 600 mg if adrenaline or felypressin is added. Plain solutions of prilocaine (0.5–1%) are specifically indicated for intravenous regional anaesthesia (Bier's block).

Bupivacaine

This is the local anaesthetic with the longest duration of action. It is also the most potent and the most toxic. It is available as 0.25%, 0.5% and 0.75% solutions and the maximum recommended dose is 2–3 mg/kg in any given 4-h period. The duration of action is 4–6 h. A hyperbaric solution (0.5%) is available for spinal anaesthesia.

Ropivacaine

It is very similar to bupivacaine but is less cardiovascularly toxic. It is also less likely to produce long-lasting motor blocks. Depending on circumstances, this can be considered an advantage or a disadvantage.

SPECIFIC LOCAL ANAESTHETIC BLOCKS

Spinal Blockade

Spinals are among the simplest yet most reliable local anaesthetic blocks to perform. The dura mater (theca) is punctured below the level at which the spinal cord usually ends (L2) and 2–3 ml of local anaesthetic is injected. Spinals are generally reserved for operations below the umbilicus, such as Caesarean section, and prostatic and hip surgery. If larger volumes of local anaesthetic are injected with the intention of performing surgery above the umbilicus, marked hypotension can occur and respiration can be compromised.

Hypotension due to sympathetically mediated vasodilatation is probably the commonest complication of spinal anaesthesia. A moderate degree of hypotension in a well-oxygenated, supine patient is of no great consequence and may well reduce operative blood loss. In conscious patients, nausea often occurs if too great a degree of hypotension is allowed to develop. Profound hypotension will result in impaired tissue perfusion with all its adverse consequences and should be treated vigorously with intravenous fluids and vasoconstrictors.

Another significant complication peculiar to spinal anaesthesia is headache. This is believed to occur because cerebrospinal fluid (CSF) continues to leak through the hole made in the dura by the initial needle puncture. Spinal headaches can be very severe and are, characteristically, postural in nature, i.e. they are relieved by lying flat and exacerbated by standing or sitting. If the headache is severe or does not rapidly settle, it should be treated with an epidural blood patch. This is performed by taking blood from the patient and injecting it aseptically into the epidural space where it clots and plugs the leak. This usually rapidly and dramatically cures the headache.

The incidence of spinal headache has been dramatically reduced in recent years by the introduction of pencil point (Sprotte or Whitacre) needles that part, rather than cut, the dural fibres, and by the development of smaller gauge needles (25g, 26g, 28g) which obviously make a smaller hole in the dura. These have enabled enthusiasts to perform spinal anaesthesia on patients who would otherwise be considered to have an unacceptably high risk of spinal headache, such as young adults and patients undergoing day-case surgery.

Small does of opiates are now frequently injected into the CSF either alone or combined with reduced amounts of local anaesthetics. These bind to receptors in the spinal cord and produce excellent analgesia with less motor, sensory and sympathetic block than local anaesthetics alone. However, opiate side-effects such as respiratory depression can occur as well as more unusual complaints such as pruritis. Respiratory depression can be reversed by naloxone without the total abolition of analgesia, whereas pruritis, if troublesome, can be relieved by antihistamines and subanaesthetic (10–20 mg) doses of propofol as well as by naloxone.

Epidural Blockade

Epidural blocks have been widely used for many years to provide pain relief during labour and it has become increasingly popular as the sole anaesthetic for operations below the umbilicus such as Caesarean section, prostatic surgery and orthopaedic surgery on the lower limbs. Epidurals are also used in conjuction with general anaesthesia for long lower-abdominal operations such as abdo-perineal resections to reduce blood pressure and hence blood loss, and to provide post-operative analgesia. Recently, epidurals have also been combined with spinals, particularly for Caesarean section, as it allows the rapid onset and dense block of a spinal to be supplemented by the ability to top-up inadequate blocks and provide post-operative analgesia via an epidural catheter.

Although effective epidural anaesthesia can be provided by a single injection into the epidural space, it is common practice to insert a catheter so that intermittant top-ups or continuous infusions of local anaesthetic can be administered. This enables anaesthesia to be maintained for long operations or analgesia to be provided into the post-operative period.

Two life threatening complications are associated with epidurals, both due to injections or infusion being inadvertently given intrathecally or intra-venously instead of into the epidural space. If a standard epidural dose of local anaesthetic (10–20 ml) is injected intrathecally, a total spinal occurs with a profound and extensive motor, sensory and sympathetic block. The patient will be unable to move, breathe or speak and marked hypotension and brady-cardia will ensue. The treatment of this potentially fatal complication is simple and logical – the hypotension is treated with fluids and vasoconstrictors, the bradycardia with atropine and the respiratory paralysis with oxygen and artificial ventilation until the block recedes.

If local anaesthetics are injected intravenously, convulsions can occur and are treated with intravenous diazepam, oxygen and assisted ventilation if necessary until the patient recovers.

Other, less-dramatic problems may also be encountered, as indicated in the following paragraphs.

Some degree of motor blockade or loss of proprioception (the ability to know where one's limbs are) may occur. If this happens, patients will be unable to move their limbs voluntarily, to stand or to walk, and will need help in altering their position.

Bladder sensation may be impaired and retention of urine can result. Micturition can sometimes be initiated by pressure over the bladder, but catheterisation may be necessary.

Owing to blockade of the sympathetic nerves, postural hypotension may occur if the patient sits or stands suddenly. All changes of position should therefore be made gradually.

The dose and concentration of local anaesthetic administered for epi-dural blockade varies with the circumstances. If motor blockade is required, 2%

NAME ....

ADDRESS ....

....

....

DATE OF BIRTH ....

HOSP. NUMBER ....

attach addressograph if available

OPERATION: ....

SPECIALTY:

ENT .... ORTHO .... TRAUMA ....

GEN SURG .... UROLOGY .... GYNAE ....

VASCULAR ...... PAEDS .... HAEMATOLOGY ....

OTHER ....

WARD .... PUMP ....

EPIDURAL INFUSION AS FOLLOWS:
(anaesthetist to complete)

BUPIVACAINE: .... ml of .... % solution

DIAMORPHINE: .... mg

(SALINE: .... ml)

TOTAL VOLUME .... ml

to run at 1 to 6 ml per hour using continuous infusion pump via epidural catheter sited at ....(insert level of insertion)

ANAESTHETIST's DETAILS:

SURNAME .... *signed* ....

date

additional patient details:

ASA GRADE: 1   2   3   4   5

WEIGHT: ....kg

DATE STARTED   .... /..... / .....

TIME STARTED   .... : ....

DATE STOPPED   .... /...../ .....

TIME STOPPED   .... : ....

TOTAL USED (ml)   ....

REASON FOR DISCONTINUATION

NO LONGER NEEDED   EPIDURAL FELL OUT

EPIDURAL SITE PROBLEM   EQUIPMENT FAILURE

OTHER ....

Comments:...

....

URINARY RETENTION (*while using EPIDURAL*)

catheter sited at operation   no catheter used

catheterised postop   in & out catheterisation

EXCESSIVE MOTOR BLOCK? yes/no ....

This patient has an epidural infusion in situ to provide continuous pain relief in the post-operative period. Analgesic agents are being infused continuously into an epidural catheter by an infusion pump at a rate prescribed by the anaesthetist. This rate may need to be increased or decreased, within the prescribed range,according to the patient's pain/sedation scores or blood pressure.

MONITORING

Patients with epidurals must have the following monitoring:

• Hourly BP and pulse rate for the duration of the epidural   • Hourly respiratory rate for the duration of the epidural

• Hourly sedation score for the duration of the epidural   • Hourly pain assessment and nausea scoring

If cathteterised, measure and record urine output 2 hourly. If < 1ml/kg/hr, inform duty H.S.

If not catheterised, check and record output 4 hourly.Look for evidence of bladder distension & if present, inform duty H.S.

SIDE EFFECTS & WHEN TO ACT OR CALL FOR HELP

Respiratory Depression

If resp. rate less than 10/min, give oxygen by mask at 4L/min & inform Pain team / duty ITU anaesthetist

If resp. rate less than 8/min, stop epidural infusion, call duty anesthetist immediately, give oxygen and get Naloxone ready.

Low Blood Pressure

If systolic bp is less than 100 mmHg, give 250ml of Saline / Hartmanns and recheck bp. If still less than 100 mmHg, call duty anaesthetist.

Urinary Retention

If patient has not p.u.'d for 4 hours or has a palpable bladder, inform duty H.S. & catheterise. (record this above).

Pruritus

Itching of the skin may occur when epidural diamorphine is used. If severe, Naloxone 0.1mg I.M. may be given.

Nausea & Vomiting

Treat in the usual way with antiemetic as prescribed on the patient's pharmacy chart.

Figure 3.4 Continuous epidural analgesia prescription

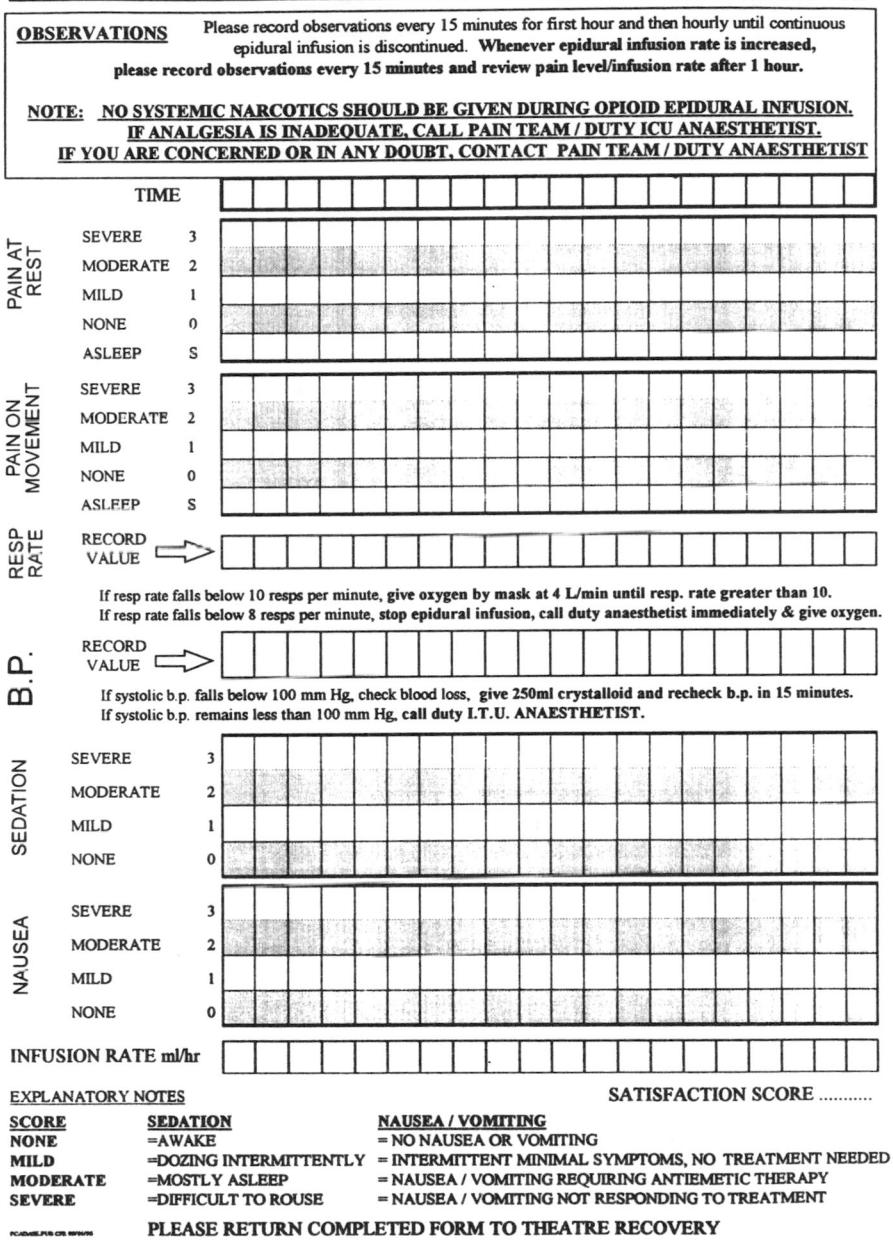

GLOUCESTERSHIRE ROYAL HOSPITAL ACUTE PAIN TEAM EPIDURAL

OBSERVATIONS Please record observations every 15 minutes for first hour and then hourly until continuous epidural infusion is discontinued. **Whenever epidural infusion rate is increased, please record observations every 15 minutes and review pain level/infusion rate after 1 hour.**

NOTE: **NO SYSTEMIC NARCOTICS SHOULD BE GIVEN DURING OPIOID EPIDURAL INFUSION.**
IF ANALGESIA IS INADEQUATE, CALL PAIN TEAM / DUTY ICU ANAESTHETIST.
IF YOU ARE CONCERNED OR IN ANY DOUBT, CONTACT PAIN TEAM / DUTY ANAESTHETIST

TIME

PAIN AT REST
SEVERE 3
MODERATE 2
MILD 1
NONE 0
ASLEEP S

PAIN ON MOVEMENT
SEVERE 3
MODERATE 2
MILD 1
NONE 0
ASLEEP S

RESP RATE
RECORD VALUE

If resp rate falls below 10 resps per minute, give oxygen by mask at 4 L/min until resp. rate greater than 10.
If resp rate falls below 8 resps per minute, stop epidural infusion, call duty anaesthetist immediately & give oxygen.

B.P.
RECORD VALUE

If systolic b.p. falls below 100 mm Hg, check blood loss, give 250ml crystalloid and recheck b.p. in 15 minutes.
If systolic b.p. remains less than 100 mm Hg, call duty I.T.U. ANAESTHETIST.

SEDATION
SEVERE 3
MODERATE 2
MILD 1
NONE 0

NAUSEA
SEVERE 3
MODERATE 2
MILD 1
NONE 0

INFUSION RATE ml/hr

EXPLANATORY NOTES   SATISFACTION SCORE ....

SCORE	SEDATION	NAUSEA / VOMITING
NONE	=AWAKE	= NO NAUSEA OR VOMITING
MILD	=DOZING INTERMITTENTLY	= INTERMITTENT MINIMAL SYMPTOMS, NO TREATMENT NEEDED
MODERATE	=MOSTLY ASLEEP	= NAUSEA / VOMITING REQUIRING ANTIEMETIC THERAPY
SEVERE	=DIFFICULT TO ROUSE	= NAUSEA / VOMITING NOT RESPONDING TO TREATMENT

PLEASE RETURN COMPLETED FORM TO THEATRE RECOVERY

Figure 3.5 Continuous epidural observation chart

lignocaine or 0.5% bupivacaine may be used. If only a sensory block is required, 1% lignocaine or 0.25% bupivacaine should be adequate. A volume of 15–25 ml or more may be injected depending on the extent of the block required. Increasing interest is being expressed in the use of continuous infusions of even lower concentrations of local anaesthetic such as 0.1% bupivacaine. These "walking" epidurals are especially popular for analgesia during labour as they allow the mother to move about freely. Sometimes, however, the analgesia they provide is inadequate but can be improved by the addition of opiates or agents such as clonidine to the infusion.

The advantages and disadvantages of adding opiates to epidural infusions of local anaesthetics are the same as those discussed when considering intrathecal opiates. The dose of opiate added is similar to that given intravenously and is approximately ten times that given intrathecally. The complications (respiratory depression, pruritis, etc) and their management are the same as when the intrathecal route is employed. Some practitioners also add clonidine to their epidural infusions as this agent is said to prolong the duration of the block and improve its quality. If the dose injected is not greater than 150 mcg, complications such as hypotension are infrequent. In our hospital, the preferred mixture is bupivacaine 0.1% (60 ml) with 5 mg diamorphine added. This is infused at 2–5 ml/h depending on the patient's requirements. Patients receiving epidural narcotics should have their vital signs and the efficacy of the infusion monitored at regular intervals.

Suitable charts for prescribing continuous epidural infusions and for monitoring patients receiving them are shown in Figures 3.4 and 3.5 (pages 58–59).

Caudal Blockade

A caudal is essentially the same as an epidural in that local anaesthetic is injected into the epidural space. The only real difference is that caudal injections are given through the sacro-coccygeal membrane where the lower two sacral vertebrae (S4–S5) have not fused in the midline rather than between two lumbar or thoracic vertebrae. Technically, caudals are easier to perform than lumbar epidurals but are only suitable for a limited range of perineal and lower abdominal operations such as circumcision, hernia repair, orchidopexy and haemorrhoidectomy.

Many of these operations are performed on children, a group on whom caudals are very easy to perform.

A suggested dose regimen using 0.25% bupivacaine would be:

- for sacral blockade   0.5 ml/kg
- for lumbar blockade   1.0 ml/kg
- for low thoracic blockade   1.25 ml/kg

Low thoracic blockade is necessary for orchidopexy operations as the testis receives its nerve supply from T10. If more than 20 ml of local anaesthetic is to be injected, it is suggested that its concentration be reduced to 0.2% by adding 1 ml of saline to every 4 ml of bupivacaine.

Although, inadvertent intrathecal or intravascular injections are theoretical complications, they are very rare. Commoner problems are urinary retention and leg weakness. If they are encountered, the child and parents should be reassured that they are normal occurences and not a cause for concern.

Local Infiltration

Frequently surgeons infiltrate wounds with long-acting local anaesthetic (bupivacaine) before they suture the skin. This is an excellent practice and contributes significantly to post-operative analgesia. Patients may still require narcotic analgesics post-operatively as they may still experience pain from bone or visceral structures.

Intercostal Nerve Blockade

Each intercostal nerve emerges through an intervertebral foramen and initially runs with an artery and vein behind the rib after which it is named. The upper six nerves innervate the chest wall, while the lower six supply the abdominal wall. Generally, the fourth nerve (T4) supplies skin at about the level of the nipple, the sixth nerve (T6) supplies skin at the level of the xiphisternum, the tenth (T10) the level of the umbilicus, and the twelfth (T12), that above the pubis.

Intercostal nerve blockade produces excellent analgesia for fractured ribs and can produce useful pain relief for most thoracic and upper abdominal incisions, particularly if they are unilateral. If the incision is in or near the midline, bilateral nerve blocks are needed, and the amount of local anaesthetic required may approach toxic levels. Although intercostal blockade usually results in an improvement in respiratory function, occasionally bilateral blockade may produce intercostal and abdominal muscle weakness and make breathing more difficult for those with chronic obstructive airways disease.

The principal complication of intercostal nerve blockade is pneumothorax but most pneumothoraces produced are small, clinically insignificant and need no treatment. However, if the patient experiences pain on breathing, starts to hyperventilate or becomes cyanosed or restless, a significant pneumothorax should be suspected. If the patient's condition allows it, a chest X-ray should be taken, but, in an emergency, a chest drain should be inserted immediately.

Tension pneumothorax requiring a chest drain is a very rare occurrence.

Intrapleural Blockade

Within the last decade, intrapleural blockade has grown in popularity for the relief of unilateral post-operative pain and, more recently, in the management of chronic pain syndromes. In this technique, the pleura is deliberately breached and a catheter inserted between the parietal and visceral layers of the pleura. Through this catheter, local anaesthetic is injected either as boluses or as a constant infusion.

The technique has proved to be exceedingly valuable for the relief of pain following unilateral thoracic and upper abdominal surgery, as well as breast and renal operations. As with intercostal blockade, pneumothorax is the commonest complication occurring in approximately 2% of patients, but, again, it is usually asymptomatic and rarely requires treatment.

Intrapleural blockade is the treatment of choice for patients with multiple fractures of ribs. It is far preferable to insert an intrapleural catheter and give top-ups through it than to attempt to perform multiple intercostal blocks every 6 hours. The usual dose of local anaesthetic injected intrapleurally is 30 ml of 0.25% bupivacaine with adrenaline. If, however, there are bilateral fractured ribs, a thoracic epidural is to be preferred as less local anaesthetic is needed, but the block is technically more difficult to perform.

Inguinal Field Blockade

Analgesia for inguinal hernia repair may be obtained by blocking the relevant nerves in the groin. This is done by injecting local anaesthetic fan-wise through the abdominal muscles medial to the iliac crest, and again, lateral to the pubic tubercle. It is wise to inject further local anaesthetic along the line of the proposed surgical incision, and again, for the surgeon to inject more local anaesthetic around the neck of the hernial sac, once it has been exposed.

Complications are few as long as excessive amounts of local anaesthetic are not used. If a long-acting agent, such as bupivacaine, is used, useful post-operative analgesia is obtained. This is a particularly valuable technique for day-case surgery and for use on frail or elderly patients. Even if a field block is not used as the sole anaesthetic, useful anlagesia can be obtained by infiltrating the line of the incision with bupivacaine.

Penile Nerve Block

This block is frequently performed in young boys undergoing circumcision or hypospadias repair. Local anaesthetic is injected around the dorsal nerves of the penis just below the pubic bone, taking care not to inject into the vascular corpora cavernosa. Further local anaesthetic should be injected subcutaneously around the base of the penis.

If intravascular injection is avoided, this block is usually without complications and provides excellent post-operative analgesia. It is imperative that adrenaline-containing solutions are not used for this block as any resulting arterial constriction would have devastating consequences!

Brachial Plexus Blockade

The brachial plexus is formed mainly from the roots of the fifth cervical to the first thoracic (C5–T1) nerves. It supplies sensation and motor power to the shoulder and arm. Although many methods of blocking the plexus have been described, three – the interscalene, supra-clavicular and axillary, are in common use.

The interscalene approach requires an injection of local anaesthetic between the scalene muscles in the neck at the level of the cricoid cartilage (C6) and the supra-clavicular, an injection above the clavicle and posterior to the subclavian artery. This latter approach, although probably likely to produce the most complete block of the brachial plexus, is also the most likely to be complicated by a pneumothorax, although the risk of this happening is slight.

As the axillary name suggests, the plexus may also be blocked in the axilla where the nerves lie in close association with the axillary artery. There is no risk of pneumothorax, but the upper nerve roots that supply the shoulder area may not be blocked.

A larger variety of upper-limb procedures can be carried out under brachial plexus blockade, but it is especially indicated in patients with chronic renal failure who need an arteriovenous shunt to be fashioned prior to dialysis. Not only does such a block avoid the risks of general anaesthesia in these ill patients, but also the vasodilatation that follows sympathetic blockade makes the surgeon's task easier.

Occasionally, a continuous brachial plexus block may be performed with a catheter inserted into the brachial plexus, usually by the axillary route. The analgesia and vasodilatation produced is especially useful in those patients who are having plastic or reconstructive surgery on the upper limb, particularly if involving microvascular anastamoses.

Patients who have had a brachial plexus block are often unaware of the position of their arm while it is anaesthetised. It is, therefore, important that during recovery, the arm is always positioned in such a way that it cannot be inadvertently injured.

Intravenous Regional Anaesthesia (Biers's Block)

At the turn of the century, Bier, a German surgeon, described an alternative method of anaesthetising the upper limb. If a tourniquet inflated to a pressure greater than systolic is placed around the upper arm and local anaesthetic solution injected intravenously in the hand, that part of the limb distal to the tourniquet will be anaesthetised. Fractures may then be reduced and minor surgery performed on the anaesthetised area.

This method of producing analgesia is much easier to perform than brachial plexus blockade, and so has become very popular. It is, however, not without its hazards, and patients can die if the block is performed by practitioners who are unaware of potential complications or their management. The most serious problems are likely to occur if the tourniquet leaks or deflates suddenly soon after the local anaesthetic had been injected. The end result is the same as if the local anaesthetic had been injected as an intravenous bolus – convulsions will rapidly occur and cardiovascular depression can follow. It is, therefore, imperative that the tourniquet is checked before use and that it is monitored constantly during the procedure. Should this misfortune happen, it is treated as discussed above with intravenous diazepam, oxygen and assisted ventilation.

Two further problems may be encountered.

Firstly, if the procedure lasts more than 20–30 min, the patient may complain of pain from the tourniquet. This is best managed by employing two tourniquets, one above the other – initially the more proximal tourniquet is inflated and the local anaesthetic injected. Once that tourniquet becomes uncomfortable, the distal cuff is inflated and the proximal cuff is deflated. Even if this two-cuff technique is used, Bier's block is not suitable for procedures likely to last more than 30–45 min.

Secondly, problems may be encountered when the tourniquet is deflated at the end of the procedure. Some local anaesthetic invariably enters the circulation, producing mild toxic effects such as ringing in the ears, a metallic taste in the mouth, or possibly dizziness or nausea. In most circumstances, the patient will need only reassurance that these symptoms are not a cause for undue concern, are transient and will quickly disappear. Their incidence can be decreased by deflating and reinflating the tourniquet a number of times, thus slowing the release of residual local anaesthetic into the circulation.

This method of local anaesthesia can also be applied to the lower limb but the volume of local anaesthetic needed is greater and the likelihood of toxic reactions is greater. Spinal or epidural blockade is generally a more sensible alternative.

Prilocaine is the drug of choice for intravenous regional anaesthesia, and usually 40 ml of 1% solution (400 mg) will produce an excellent upper limb block. Lignocaine can also be used but its therapeutic index is less and the likelihood of side-effects is greater. Bupivacaine must never be used, as it is far too toxic for intravenous injection.

Digital Nerve Blockade

Individual digits, be they fingers or toes, can easily be blocked by injecting small volumes of local anaesthetic into the web space on either side of the digit where the digital nerves run, or in a weal around the medial aspect of the thumb or great toe. Foreign bodies or in-growing toe nails can then be painlessly removed or lacerations sutured.

As the digits are supplied by end-arteries, adrenaline-containing solutions must never be used for digital nerve blockade in case ischaemic gangrene results.

Femoral Nerve Blockade

This is probably the most useful block that can be performed on the leg. The femoral nerve lies lateral to the femoral artery as they both pass beneath the inguinal ligament and enter the thigh. An isolated femoral nerve block produces an area of analgesia on the anterior aspect of the thigh, but, more importantly, can relieve the pain of a fractured shaft of femur.

If a larger volume (20–30 ml) of local anaesthetic is injected, it will track upwards in the same fascial plane as the femoral nerve and block the obturator and lateral cutaneous nerves as well, so producing the so-called 3:1 block. Such a block is especially indicated when split skin grafts are taken from the anterolateral aspect of the thigh. The donor site can be extremely painful but will be rendered totally pain-free by this block. It is also a useful block for relieving anterior knee pain following total knee replacement.

PATIENT MANAGEMENT IN THE PACU

Most of the specific complications of local anaesthetic blocks have been mentioned above. They generally occur as, or, soon after the local anaesthetic is injected, and therefore are not usually seen in the PACU.

A number of potentially major complications may, however, be encountered by PACU staff:

1. If catheters have been inserted into the epidural space, they can migrate into either the intrathecal space (CSF) or intravascularly. If a further top-up is given in the PACU, either a total spinal (following a CSF injection) or a grand mal convulsion (following an intravenous injection) could occur. In most cases, aspiration of the catheter prior to injection should reveal either CSF or blood if migration has occurred.

2. All injections through catheters should be given by personnel who are able to recognise potential complications and manage them appropriately.

3. Patients who have had major blocks (epidurals and spinals) may have significant residual sympathetic block even if motor and sensory blocks have regressed. This can result in hypotension or fainting if they are allowed to sit up or stand. All changes in position should be made slowly so that hypotension can be identified before it causes significant problems.

4. Any area of residual sensory block should be identified. In the absence of normal sensation, patients can inadvertently injure such areas without appreciating it. Both the patient and ward staff should be reminded to exercise due care.

5. It is self-evident that when a patient is transferred to the care of ward staff, the latter are informed if a local anaesthetic block has been performed and the degree to which the patient is still affected by the block. They may need to be told about potential problems associated with the block, especially if they do not regularly care for patients who receive local anaesthetic blocks.

References and Bibliography

Cousins MJ, Bridenbaugh PO (1988). Neural Blockade in Clinical Anaesthesia and the Management of Pain, 2nd edn. Lippincott, Philadelphia.

Cousins MJ, Philips GD (1986). Acute Pain Management. Churchill Livingstone, London.

Diamond AW, Coniam SW (1996). The Management of Chronic Pain, 2nd edn. Oxford Medical Publications, Oxford.

Melzack R, Wall PD (1965). Pain mechanisms: a new theory. Science, 150, 971-979.

Melzack R, Wall PD (1989). Textbook of Pain. Churchill Livingstone, London.

Wildsmith JAW, Armitage EN (1987). Principles and Practice of Regional Anaesthesia. Churchill Livingstone, London.

Chapter 4
COMPLICATIONS

RESPIRATORY COMPLICATIONS

The function of the respiratory system is the delivery of oxygen to, and the elimination of carbon dioxide from, the blood. Any respiratory complication will, if uncorrected, lead to inadequate oxygenation (hypoxaemia) and/or retention of CO_2 (hypercarbia), and these conditions must be readily recognised by recovery staff. The incidence of such problems is greater after lengthy anaesthesia and surgery.

Signs of Hypoxaemia

1. Cyanosis. This may be difficult to detect in the presence of anaemia or poor peripheral perfusion. Reduced oxygen saturation is displayed on the oximeter.
2. Restlessness and confusion. This indicates impaired cerebral oxygenation.
3. Tachycardia followed by bradycardia.

Signs of Hypercarbia

1. Tachycardia.
2. Hypertension.
3. Sweating.
4. Irregular pulse, especially *pulsus bigeminus.*
5. Flushed skin owing to capillary vasodilation. (This may give a mistaken impression of well-being.)
6. Clouding of consciousness.

The routine use of pulse oximeters is recommended as it allows hypoxaemia to be recognised early, before cyanosis develops. The diagnosis may be confirmed by taking a sample of arterial blood for blood gas analysis.

Upper Airway Obstruction

Indications of Partial Obstruction of the Airway

1. Stertorous breathing, i.e. snoring.
2. Inspiratory stridor, i.e. a crowing noise on inspiration.
3. Laboured breathing. Use of the accessory muscles of respiration (sterno-mastoids, scalenes) with retraction of the head on inspiration and flaring of the nostrils.
4. Rocking movements of the abdomen and chest. Instead of the abdomen and chest rising and falling in phase together, downward descent of the diaphragm with abdominal distension is accompanied by retraction or indrawing of the thorax, creating a see-saw or rocking motion of the chest and abdomen (external paradoxical respiration). This becomes more marked as the degree of obstruction increases.

Signs of Complete Respiratory Obstruction

1. No movement of air is detectable at the airway.
2. There are no breath sounds.
3. Signs of hypoxia rapidly develop.
4. Dysrhythmias and bradycardia occur.

It is important to note that movements of the chest are not synonymous with a clear airway; indeed, excessive chest movements may occur in the presence of complete airway obstruction. Remember also that although partial obstruction is accompanied by noisy respiration, total obstruction is silent.

Causes

1. *Tongue.* In the unconscious patient with the jaw relaxed the tongue may fall back and obstruct the airway.
2. *Foreign material in the pharynx:*
   (a) Excess mucus or saliva.
   (b) Gastric contents from vomiting or regurgitation.
   (c) Blood following oral or nasal surgery.
   (d) Broken or dislodged teeth.
   (e) Dental packs not removed at extubation.
3. *Laryngospasm,* resulting from stimulation of the larynx during emergence from anaesthesia. This may be caused by foreign material (as above) or by clumsy extubation or suction.

The following are less common but nevertheless potentially lethal:

4. *Laryngeal oedema* following trauma, intubation or infection. This is especially dangerous in the young, when the airway is of narrow diameter, and in patients with pre-eclamptic toxaemia who are prone to oedema.
5. *External pressure on the trachea:*
    (a) Haematoma following thyroid surgery or following attempts at internal jugular cannulation.
    (b) Use of constrictive Elastoplast bandages.
6. *Abductor paralysis of vocal cords.* This may occur following damage to the recurrent laryngeal nerve during thyroid surgery (see page 123).
7. *Tracheal collapse* following thyroidectomy.

Management

1. Extend the neck.
2. Lift the jaw forward.
3. Insert an oral airway. If the teeth are tightly clenched owing to spasm of the masseters, firm downward pressure on the mandible may be necessary to enable the airway to be inserted. If this fails, a nasopharyngeal airway may be inserted to bypass the obstruction. If the obstruction remains unrelieved, foreign material in the pharynx must be suspected. If the patient is not already on his side then:
4. Turn the patient on to his side (preferably the left, in case subsequent laryngoscopy becomes necessary).
5. Tilt the head down (Trendelenburg position) to help clear any foreign material.
6. Apply suction to pharynx with a rigid Yankauer sucker or a large suction catheter.

If these measures are unsuccessful proceed to:

7. Laryngoscopy – so that foreign material can be sucked out under direct vision or removed using Magill forceps. If the larynx is clear but the vocal cords are in spasm:
8. Give oxygen by anaesthetic face mask and Mapleson C circuit (Figure 2.14). Apply gentle pressure to the reservoir bag to try to overcome the spasm. If this is unsuccessful, give intravenous suxamethonium (succinylcholine) to relax the cords and ventilate the lungs. Endotracheal intubation may be necessary.

Laryngeal Oedema

Although this usually resolves spontaneously, preparations for rapid intubation should be made. The following may aid spontaneous resolution:

(a) Head-up position to improve venous drainage.
(b) Humidification.
(c) Steroids.
(d) Diuretics.
(e) Inhalation of nebulised adrenaline (racemic epinephrine).

The inhalation of a mixture of helium 80% and oxygen 20% will reduce the resistance to air flow and make breathing easier.

External Pressure on the Trachea
Abductor Paralysis of Vocal Cords
Tracheal Collapse
} See Complications of Thyroid Surgery (page 123)

Cricothyrotomy

In the event of a complete obstruction of the upper airway which cannot be resolved by the above measures, an emergency cricothyrotomy may be required. The cricothyrotomy needle is inserted through the cricothyroid membrane into the trachea to bypass the obstruction. If a cricothyrotomy set is unavailable any large (14 G) intravenous cannula can be used, but it must be connected to a high-pressure source of oxygen to overcome the resistance to air flow.

Inadequate Ventilation (Hypoventilation)

If correction of upper-airway obstruction does not lead to the resumption of a normal breathing pattern or if signs of hypoxaemia or hypercarbia develop, then inadequate alveolar ventilation must be suspected. Confirmation can be obtained by:

1. *Measuring the respiratory minute volume,* using a Wright's spirometer (normal values should exceed 5 litres/min). Because of the difficulty of obtaining an airtight fit with a mask, this method may be unsatisfactory in patients who are not intubated.
2. *Analysing blood gases* on an arterial sample. Inadequate alveolar ventilation is characterised by a respiratory acidosis (pH < 7.35, $PaCO_2 > 6$ kPa).

Except in an emergency, when intubation and controlled ventilation must be instituted without delay, an attempt should be made to determine the cause of the inadequate ventilation so that specific treatment aimed at correcting this may be undertaken.

Causes

Causes of inadequate ventilation in the immediate post-operative period are:

1. Depression of the respiratory centre/Cheyne–Stokes respiration.
2. Residual muscle paralysis.
3. Interference with the mechanics of respiration.

Depression of Respiratory Centre

Depression of the respiratory centre may be due to:

1. Drugs:
   (a) Opiates given before or during anaesthesia.
   (b) Barbiturates.
   (c) Inhalation agents.
2. Lack of respiratory drive:
   (a) Low $PaCO_2$ following hyperventilation during anaesthesia.
   (b) Loss of hypoxic drive owing to administrations of high concentrations of oxygen to patients suffering from chronic pulmonary disease.

Central depression may be suspected by:

1. Delayed return of consciousness. Patients should normally show signs of returning consciousness within 15 min of arrival in the recovery room.
2. Respiratory rate below 10 breaths/min with a low tidal volume.
3. Constricted pupils following opiate administration.
4. History of chronic pulmonary disease.

Management

If central depression owing to opiates is suspected, this may be corrected by either of the following:

1. Intravenous naloxone, 0.1–0.4 mg. This drug is a specific opiate antagonist and is therefore ineffective in other forms of respiratory depression. It should be given slowly in increments of 0.1 mg every 2–3 min and its effect titrated against the patient's respiratory response. Excessive doses will reverse not only the respiratory depression but also the analgesic effect of the opiates, causing the patient unnecessary pain. To extend the duration of action, subsequent injections can be given by the intramuscular route.
2. Intravenous doxapram, 1 mg/kg. This drug is a direct stimulant of the respiratory centre and has advantages over naloxone as it is effective for other causes of central respiratory depression and does not reverse analgesia.

Since the depressant effects of the opiates may outlast either of these antidotes, they may have to be repeated.

If there is a history of pulmonary disease, graded concentrations of oxygen should be given using a Venturi mask and progress monitored by repeated blood gas analysis.

If the situation does not improve, it is safer to intubate the trachea and electively ventilate the lungs until the effects of anaesthesia and surgery have worn off.

Cheyne–Stokes Respiration

This is an irregular pattern of respiration characterised by periods of hyperventilation alternating with hypoventilation. It is more commonly seen in elderly patients. Causes of Cheyne–Stokes respiration are:

1. Left ventricular failure.
2. Depression of respiratory centre.
3. Raised intracranial pressure.
4. Uraemia.

Management

This condition may be aggravated by the administration of sedative drugs which should be used with caution in the recovery period.

An underlying condition should be sought and treated if possible. If respiration becomes inadequate, intubation and controlled ventilation will be required.

Residual Paralysis

Residual paralysis may be due to the continued action of muscle relaxants given during anaesthesia causing neuromuscular block of either the depolarising or non-depolarising type. Residual paralysis should be suspected if there is:

1. Laboured breathing – use of accessory muscles of respiration (extension of the neck on inspiration).
2. Rapid shallow breathing with minimal chest movement.
3. Flaring of the nostrils and/or raising of the eyebrows.
4. Unexplained restlessness.
5. Attempts to speak. The patient may say that they cannot breathe properly.
6. Tracheal tug (downward movement of trachea and thyroid cartilage on inspiration).

Simple Bedside Tests to Indicate Residual Paralysis

1. Ask the patient to grip your hand, or to raise his head from the pillow, or protrude his tongue for several seconds.
2. Measure the vital capacity – normal value should exceed 50 ml/kg.

The type of treatment will depend on whether the residual paralysis is due to depolarising (phase I) or non-depolarising (phase II) block. A knowledge of type, quantity and timing of the muscle relaxants given during anaesthesia will usually clarify this, but if doubt remains additional information may be obtained from:

1. *Peripheral nerve stimulation.* If a train of four supramaximal stimuli at a frequency of 2 Hz is applied to the ulnar nerve, contraction of the hand muscles will result. This is painful for the conscious patient and should not be applied more frequently than is essential. Fade with successive stimuli confirms non-depolarising block. Significant paralysis is indicated if the ratio of the fourth to the first response is less than 50%.
2. *Edrophonium test.* An intravenous injection of the short-acting anticholinesterase drug edrophonium will increase muscle strength if the patient has a non-depolarising block. It is unwise to use the longer-acting neostigmine as it will exacerbate a depolarising block.

Depolarising Block (Phase I Block)

Suxamethonium (succinylcholine) is normally metabolised by cholinesterase in the blood within 5–10 min of administration with the resumption of spontaneous respiration. Paralysis is prolonged in the presence of:

1. *Abnormal cholinesterase.* A rare inherited condition in which there is an impaired ability to metabolise suxamethonium.
2. *Reduced amounts of cholinesterase.* Cholinesterase is synthesised in the liver and may be deficient in liver disease or malnutrition.
3. *Concurrent administration of anticholinesterases*, e.g. ecothiopate (phospholine iodide) used in the treatment of glaucoma.

Management of Phase I Block

If, following the administration of suxamethonium (succinylcholine), spontaneous respiration has not returned by the time the patient arrives in the recovery unit, assisted ventilation must be continued. Spontaneous respiration is normally resumed within 2 h but can be expedited by the administration of cholinesterase in the form of fresh frozen plasma.

Before the patient finally leaves hospital, blood should be taken for estimation of cholinesterase level and dibucaine number to confirm the cause. If abnormal cholinesterase is demonstrated by a low dibucaine number (normal 80%), the family practitioner must be notified and other members of the family investigated as they may also be affected.

Non-depolarising Block (Phase II Block)

Non-depolarising block may be due to:

1. *Excessive administration of non-depolarising relaxants* in relation to the patient's size and the duration of surgery. During hypothermia there is resistance to the non-depolarising relaxants and large quantities are required to produce a block. On re-warming, signs of overdose may become apparent when normal sensitivity is restored.
2. *Sensitivity to relaxants*, e.g. in patients with myasthenia gravis.
3. *Potentiation of relaxants* owing to:
   (a) Hypokalaemia (diuretic therapy, prolonged pre-operative bowel wash-out).
   (b) Acidosis (vomiting, blood transfusion, hypotension).
   (c) Administration of large quantities of antibiotics, especially strepto-mycin and related aminoglycosides, e.g. polymyxins, tetracycline, lincomycin.
   (d) Hypocalaemia.
4. *Impaired excretion or metabolism of relaxants* (kidney or liver disease).
5. *Excessive administration of depolarising relaxants.* When the amount of suxamethonium (succinylcholine) administered exceeds 300 mg the de-polarising block (phase I) may develop into a non-depolarising (phase II) block.

Management of Phase II Block

1. Administer intravenous neostigmine (preceded by atropine or, if there is tachycardia, glycopyronium to a total dose, including that given at the end of surgery, of 0.08 mg/kg. If this does not reverse the neuromuscular block, controlled ventilation is continued while further attempts are made to determine the cause. Care should be taken to administer further anaesthesia if consciousness returns.
2. Take blood for blood gas and electrolyte estimation.
3. Correct metabolic acidosis with intravenous sodium bicarbonate using the formula – Base deficit × Body weight (in kg) × $\frac{1}{3}$ = Amount (mmol) of sodium bicarbonate required. This is normally given in smaller increments and the effect measured by serial blood gas estimations.
4. Correct hypokalaemia by intravenous potassium chloride. Up to 20 mmol of a dilute solution may be given per hour under continuous ECG monitor-ing.
5. If hypocalcaemia is suspected following massive transfusion of stored blood

or if large quantities of antibiotics have been given, 10 ml of 10% calcium chloride intravenously may correct the situation.

Conditions Affecting the Mechanics of Respiration

Inadequate ventilation may occur post-operatively if respiratory movements are impaired by:

1. Pain from a high abdominal or thoracic incision.
2. Obesity (page 160).
3. Tight abdominal or thoracic strapping.
4. Pneumothorax or haemothorax.

Management

1. Give oxygen by face mask to increase the inspired oxygen concentration (F_iO_2).
2. Sit the patient up to lessen the pressure on the diaphragm.
3. Ensure adequate analgesia.
4. Encourage deep breathing by means of physiotherapy.

If the history or clinical findings suggest pneumothorax or haemothorax, an X-ray of the chest should be taken and appropriate management instituted (page 78).

Progress can be monitored by serial blood gas estimation. If there is no improvement with the above measures, intubation and controlled ventilation will be required.

Hypoxaemia

Causes

In addition to the hypoxaemia resulting from generalised underventilation of the lungs and a reduced respiratory minute volume (page 70), it may also be caused post-operatively by the following:

1. *Diffusion hypoxaemia* (Fink effect). In the first few minutes after nitrous oxide is discontinued, it comes out of solution in the blood and diffuses into the alveoli. The concentration of oxygen is, therefore, reduced below normal if the patient is breathing room air. Oxygen should always be administered after nitrous oxide is discontinued.
2. *Increased oxygen utilisation* accompanying shivering, convulsions, pyrexia, thyroid crisis.

3. *Ventilation perfusion (V:Q) imbalance* caused by regional underventilation. Some alveoli continue to receive a normal blood supply but are not adequately ventilated. This occurs if there is atelectasis due to:
   (a) Absorption collapse distal to an obstruction caused by plugs of mucus or inhalation of foreign material.
   (b) Surgical compression of the lung during thoracotomy.
   (c) Airway closure at the bases owing to restricted movements because of pain.
   (d) Pneumonia.
   (e) Pulmonary oedema.

Management

1. Administer oxygen by face mask to increase the proportion of inspired oxygen (F_iO_2). This is particularly important in the elderly and in those with a reduced cardiopulmonary reserve.

   If atelectasis is the likely cause:

2. Encourage deep breathing and arrange regular physiotherapy.
3. Ensure there is adequate analgesia.
4. Monitor progress by oximetry and blood gas estimations.

Bronchospasm

In spontaneously breathing patients, bronchospasm is characterised by dyspnoea and wheezing, especially during expiration. In patients being ventilated, an increased airway pressure is required to inflate the lungs (decreased compliance).

Causes

1. *Predominance of parasympathetic tone*, e.g. following neostigmine or β-blockers such as propranolol or esmolol.
2. *Irritation of the larynx* during emergence from anaesthesia, e.g. by secretions, gastric contents, endotracheal tube, suction catheter. Chronic bronchitics and smokers are especially prone to this problem.
3. *Anaphylactoid reactions* owing to histamine release following administration of drugs such as *d*-tubocurarine, Haemaccel, NSAIDs or following blood transfusions.
4. *Asthma.*

Management

1. Administration of oxygen.
2. Bronchodilators, e.g. aminophylline 250–500 mg intravenously given slowly to minimise tachycardia *or* salbutamol (albuterol) either intravenously or via a nebuliser (see Figure 4.1).
3. Hydrocortisone 100 mg i.v. to reduce mucosal swelling.

   If bronchospasm and dyspnoea persist despite these measures:

4. Intubate and ventilate the lungs.

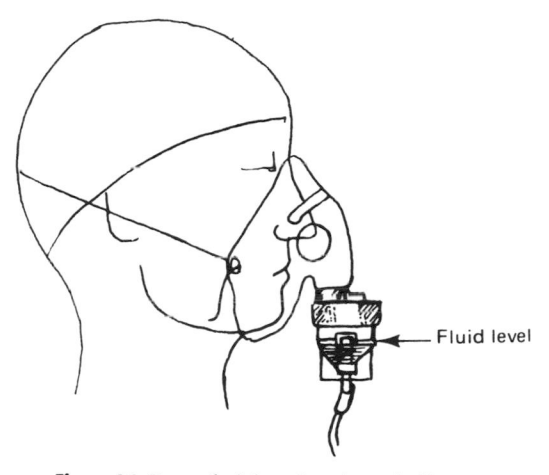

Figure 4.1 Drug administration via a nebuliser

Aspiration of Gastric Contents

During recovery from general anaesthesia the laryngeal reflex may be depressed. Therefore, if vomiting or regurgitation occurs, the gastric contents may be aspirated into the trachea and lungs. To reduce this risk, patients recovering from anaesthesia are normally nursed on their sides so that regurgitated gastric contents do not pool in the posterior pharynx, but are cleared with the aid of gravity.

If Vomiting Occurs During the Recovery Period:

1. *Turn the patient onto his side,* if not already in this position. The left side is preferable since if the patient is supine, inhaled material may normally enter the right lung and drainage will be facilitated with this lung uppermost. In addition, subsequent laryngoscopy is easiest with the patient on the left side.
2. *Tilt the bed head down* (Trendelenburg position).

3. *Apply suction to the pharynx.* Laryngoscopy and Magill forceps may be required to remove solid material.
4. *Give oxygen by face mask.*

If Aspiration Has Occurred:

5. *Intubate* and give 100% oxygen.
6. *Apply suction* to the trachea and main bronchi using a fine catheter via the endotracheal tube.
7. *Consider bronchoscopy* if hypoxia persists or if solid material has been inhaled.
8. *Give bronchodilators* as required to relieve bronchospasm (see page 76).
9. *Administer hydrocortisone* 100–500 mg i.v. to reduce mucosal swelling.
10. *Encourage coughing* and arrange vigorous physiotherapy in an attempt to clear the lungs.

Antibiotics are not usually recommended at this stage, as gastric contents are usually sterile, but may be added if pyrexia develops or when the results of sputum culture become known. An early X-ray of the chest may provide a baseline for subsequent comparison.

Chemical Pneumonitis (Mendelson's Syndrome)

If the gastric contents are highly acid (pH < 2.5), as may occur during labour, aspiration into the lung may also cause chemical pneumonitis.

Aspiration of a small volume of acidic gastric contents may be silent and the signs of chemical pneumonitis may not develop for several hours. It must be suspected if a patient develops tachypnoea, cyanosis, tachycardia and wheezing in the recovery period. The chest X-ray may show diffuse opacities over the affected area, often the right base, thus confirming the diagnosis.

These patients should be transferred to an intensive-care unit for management as severe respiratory difficulties may subsequently occur. The recovery-room nurse must always record suspected regurgitation and vomiting.

Pneumothorax and Haemothorax

Pneumothorax (the presence of air in the pleural cavity) may become evident during recovery from anaesthesia. It is suggested by:

1. Chest pain.
2. Dyspnoea.
3. Cyanosis.
4. Diminished air entry on the affected side.

A chest X-ray will confirm the diagnosis.

Causes

1. Damage to pleura following surgery or trauma.
2. Accidental pleural puncture following intercostal nerve block or supra-clavicular brachial plexus block, or during attempts at internal jugular or subclavian vein cannulation.
3. Alveolar rupture during intermittent positive-pressure ventilation or the spontaneous rupture of an emphysematous bulla.

Management

A small pneumothorax unaccompanied by clinical features may resolve spontaneously and not require treatment.

A larger pneumothorax requires the insertion of a chest drain with under-water seal. A suitable site is the second interspace in the mid-clavicular line.

N.B. The administration of nitrous oxide in the presence of a pneumothorax will increase its size and should be avoided.

If the chest X-ray demonstrates the presence of fluid in the pleural cavity (haemothorax, pleural effusion), this should be released by a chest drain placed in the eighth space in the posterior axillary line.

Tension Pneumothorax

If the pneumothorax is under tension, the signs will be more acute. In addition there will be:

1. Cardiovascular collapse owing to diminished venous return.
2. Deviation of the trachea and displacement of the apex beat away from the affected side.
3. Increasing difficulty in inflating the lungs in the ventilated patient.

Management

Urgent insertion of a chest drain (see page 131). In an emergency, the increased intrapleural pressure can be reduced rapidly by inserting a large-bore intravenous cannula into the second intercostal space while equipment is prepared for a more formal procedure.

CARDIOVASCULAR COMPLICATIONS

Hypotension

The post-operative blood pressure should not be considered in isolation, but as part of a trend, and interpreted in relation to the pulse rate and to other findings such as the pre-operative value and the state of the peripheral perfusion. For example, a reduction of 30 mmHg in the systolic pressure of a hypertensive patient may be a significant fall yet still be within the normal range. On the other hand, in the presence of good peripheral perfusion, a blood pressure below the normal range may be satisfactory following certain anaesthetic techniques (page 145).

A reduced blood pressure is frequently due to the continuing action of drugs used during anaesthesia (Table 4.1) and will usually revert to normal as the agents are eliminated. While patients are recovering from the effects of these agents, vasomotor tone may be impaired and with it the patient's ability to compensate for sudden changes in posture. A temporary fall in blood pressure may follow transfer of the patient from the operating table or the lowering of the legs from the lithotomy position, and the patient should not sit up until the effects of these agents have worn off.

If, on admission to the recovery unit, the systolic blood pressure is below 100 mmHg, the patient's progress should be monitored carefully until normal values are restored. If peripheral perfusion is impaired, hypovolaemia and diminished cardiac output must be excluded.

Table 4.1. Drugs used during anaesthesia causing hypotension

1. *Myocardial depression*
   Inhalational anaesthetic agents, e.g. halothane, enflurane
   β-blocking agents, e.g. propranolol, labetalol
   Intravenous induction agents, e.g. thiopentone, propofol
2. *Diminished peripheral vascular resistance*
   Inhalational anaesthetic agents, e.g. isoflurane
   Sympathetic blockade:
      (a) Ganglion-blocking agents, e.g. trimetaphan
      (b) Local anaesthetic agents used for spinal or epidural anaesthesia
3. *Vasodilating drugs:* nitroglycerine, nitroprusside, chlorpromazine, droperidol, opiates

Hypovolaemia

Hypotension and poor peripheral perfusion are accompanied by increasing heart rate, pallor, collapsed veins (a low central venous pressure reading will confirm this) and oliguria (urine output < 0.5ml/(kg h).

Causes

1. Inadequate fluid replacement following pre-operative dehydration or prolonged surgery with bowel exposure.
2. Inadequate replacement of blood.

Management

1. Give oxygen by face mask to increase the percentage of oxygen inspired (F_iO_2).
2. Elevate the foot of the bed.
3. Increase the rate of intravenous infusion.

N.B. Vasoconstricting agents are not recommended in the presence of hypovolaemia since they will further decrease tissue perfusion.

If there has been haemorrhage, a blood transfusion may be necessary. Until cross-matched blood is ready, the following substitutes may be used:

1. Modified gelatins (Haemaccel or Gelofusin).
2. Modified starch solutions (Hespan or Haesteril).
3. Human plasma protein fraction (HPPF).
4. Human albumin solution (HAS).

If hypotension, pallor and collapsed veins persist despite these measures, then continued bleeding must be suspected. This may be either:

1. *Revealed*, e.g. blood in drainage bottles, bladder irrigation or on dressings and packs.
2. *Concealed*, e.g. intra-abdominal.

In either case the transfusion must be continued and the surgeon and anaesthetist notified as further surgery may be required. Alternatively, persistent bleeding may be due to a failure of coagulation and this may be suspected if a sample of blood in a plain tube does not clot within 10 min (see page 108). Blood should then be taken for a formal coagulation screen.

Diminished Cardiac Output

If hypotension and poor peripheral perfusion are not due to hypovolaemia then a diminished cardiac output must be considered. This may be indicated by distended veins, a raised CVP and a falling pulse pressure. The last is the difference between the systolic and diastolic pressure and is normally about 40 mmHg.

Causes and Management

1. *Cardiac failure.* A review of the patient's previous medical history and the intra-operative fluid balance may suggest this possibility. Breathlessness, tachycardia and pulmonary and peripheral oedema may confirm it.
   Management will include:
   (a) Oxygen therapy.
   (b) Posture (reverse Trendelenburg position).
   (c) Diuretics.

   (d) Fluid restriction.
   (e) Inotropic support (dopamine, dobutamine, digoxin).
   (f) Intubation and intermittent positive-pressure ventilation (in extreme cases only).

2. *Myocardial infarction.* There may be history of myocardial ischaemia or the classical description of chest pain may be present. However, infarction can occur silently in patients with no previous history of cardiac disease. A 12-lead ECG should be performed and blood taken for enzyme studies. Although these may not contribute to the immediate management of the patient, they may provide a valuable baseline for future reference.

3. *Pulmonary embolus.* Although this is uncommon in the immediate post-operative period, pleuritic chest pain and haemoptysis may suggest this diagnosis. A chest X-ray and full ECG should be obtained. Treatment includes oxygen therapy, pain relief and heparinisation.

4. *Cardiac tamponade.* This may follow surgery or trauma in the region of the mediastinum or, rarely, perforation of the myocardium by a central venous or pulmonary artery catheter. Faint heart sounds and a rising CVP accompanied by a falling blood pressure may suggest this possibility. Widening of the mediastinum on chest X-ray will provide confirmation. Emergency treatment is by needle aspiration from below the xiphisternum, but a formal thoracotomy may be necessary.

5. *Tension pneumothorax* (see page 79).

Other Causes of Hypotension

If hypovolaemia and diminished cardiac output have been excluded, and the cause of hypotension remains obscure, the following should be considered:

1. *Septicaemia.* Especially following bowel or urological surgery. This may be suspected by pyrexia, tachycardia, flushing, sweating or delirium. Management includes vigorous intravenous therapy to achieve and maintain normal venous pressure, and inotropic, antibiotic and steroid therapy.

2. *Inadequate steroid cover.* For patients on long-term steroid therapy or with undiagnosed Addison's disease. Initial management will consist of fluid replacement and steroid therapy (page 147).

3. *Mismatched blood transfusion.* Hypotension may accompany other signs of mismatched transfusion, such as pyrexia, urticaria, flushing, shivering, haematuria and persistent bleeding. The transfusion should be stopped immediately and samples of the transfused blood and patient's blood sent to the laboratory for further investigations (see page 108).

4. *Pain.* Usually causes hypertension but hypotension is sometimes seen and may respond to the administration of analgesics.

Hypertension

Like pre-operative hypertension, this is not uncommon in the immediate post-operative period

Causes

1. Pain.
2. Distension of bladder.
3. Respiratory depression with hypercarbia.
4. Overtransfusion.
5. Cardiovascular surgery.
6. Drugs used during anaesthesia, e.g. ketamine, methoxamine, ephedrine.
7. Underlying condition, e.g. phaeochromocytoma, hyperthyroidism, raised intra-cranial pressure, pre-eclamptic toxaemia.

Management

Once pain, bladder distension and respiratory complications have been treated, the hypertension usually reverts to normal within 2h without the need for specific treatment. However, in those with coronary artery or cerebrovascular disease, excessive hypertension may cause myocardial ischaemia or cerebral haemorrhage and active management is required. Similarly, following vascular surgery hypertension will cause an unnecessary strain on the graft and should be avoided.

Numerous drugs are available to reduce blood pressure, for example:

1. α-Blocking agents, e.g. phentolamine, chlorpromazine.
2. Ganglion-blocking agents, e.g. trimetaphan.
3. Drugs acting directly on peripheral vessels, e.g. sodium nitroprusside, nitroglycerine, hydralazine, nifedipine.

In the presence of an accompanying tachycardia a combined α- and β-blocking agent such as labetalol may be useful.

It is important to exclude any of the underlying conditions which will require specific treatment, although in 30% of the patients no obvious cause can be found.

Bradycardia

Sinus Bradycardia

A heart rate of less than 60 per minute is normal in fit athletes but may signify an underlying condition requiring correction.

Causes

1. Continuing action of drugs used before or during anaesthesia, e.g. opiates, neostigmine, β-blocking agents (even when used as eye-drops), digoxin.
2. High sympathetic blockade following spinal or epidural anaesthesia.
3. Parasympathetic stimulation due to pain or pharyngeal suction.
4. Hypoxia.
5. Raised intracranial pressure.
6. Decreased metabolic rate due to hypothermia, hypothyroidism.
7. Acute gastric dilatation.

Management

Intravenous atropine (0.5–2 mg) will usually correct any excessive parasympathetic tone or, alternatively, ephedrine may be used if there is an accompanying sympathetic blockade with hypotension.

If there is no response and hypoxia and raised intracranial pressure can be excluded, an ECG is required to differentiate between sinus bradycardia and heart block. In sinus bradycardia the PR interval is normal, i.e. less than 0.2 s (Figure 4.2).

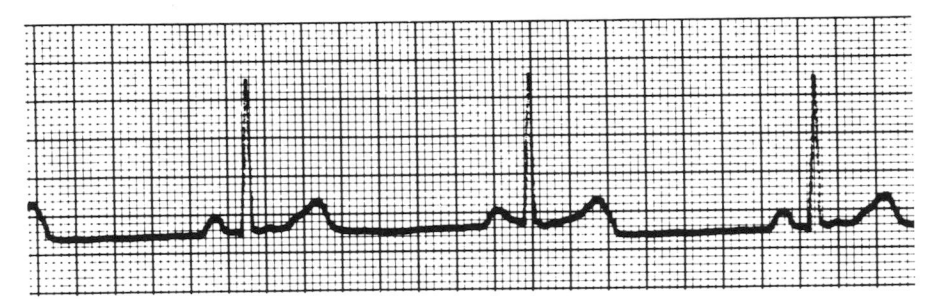

Figure 4.2 Sinus bradycardia

Heart Block

Three types of heart block are identified on ECG:

First-degree heart block: PR interval greater than 0.2 s.

Second-degree heart block:

> Mobitz type I (Wenckebach phenomenon). Gradual lengthening of PR interval until a dropped beat occurs.
>
> Mobitz type II. There is a failure of conduction so that only every second or third atrial impulse is conducted to the ventricles (2:1 or 3:1 block).

Third-degree heart block: Complete AV dissociation. No atrial impulses are conducted to the ventricles, which beat independently at a slow rate (Figure 4.3).

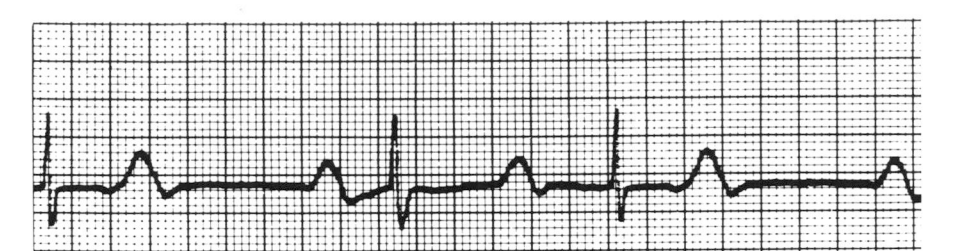

Figure 4.3 Third-degree heart block

Causes

1. Myocardial infarction.
2. Drugs depressing myocardial conduction, e.g. digitalis, disopyramide, β-blocking agents.

Management

Symptoms due to heart block, e.g. dizziness, fainting and poor peripheral perfusion, can frequently be treated by the infusion of a dilute solution of isoprenaline (isoproterenol) 4 mg in 500 ml 5% dextrose given via a paediatric infusion set. If this fails, a pacemaker must be inserted.

Tachycardia

Sinus Tachycardia

There is a normal sinus rhythm but with a rate of over 100/min.

A tachycardia is normal in infants and small children. Rates of up to 150/min are well tolerated in patients with normal cardiac function and seldom require treatment, but problems may arise in those with underlying heart disease because of the increased myocardial oxygen consumption and diminished stroke volume.

Causes

1. Pain
2. Respiratory problems causing hypercarbia or hypoxia.
3. Circulatory disturbance, e.g. hypocalcaemia, hypervolaemia.
4. Infection.
5. Drugs, e.g. atropine, ephedrine, adrenaline (epinephrine), ketamine.
6. Anxiety.
7. Underlying conditions, e.g. hyperthyroidism, phaeochromocytoma.

Management

This consists of treatment of the underlying cause:

1. Administer analgesics as required to relieve pain.
2. Assess respiratory function using blood-gas analysis if necessary. For treatment of inadequate ventilation, see pages 70–79.
3. Assess circulation for signs of hypovolaemia or hypervolaemia.
   (a) *Hypovolaemia:* cold clammy skin, thready pulse, collapsed veins, hypotension. Treat by fluid replacement.
   (b) *Hypervolaemia:* strong pulse, distended veins, normal or high blood pressure. Treat by fluid restriction, diuretics.
4. Give reassurance and add anxiolytics as required.

Supraventricular and Ventricular Tachycardia (SVT and VT)

A heart rate in the region of 150–250/min suggests either supraventricular or ventricular tachycardia. These may be accompanied by dizziness, palpitations, angina or chest pain and, if untreated, may lead to circulatory failure.

Causes

1. Hypoxia.
2. Hypercarbia.
3. Electrolyte disturbance, especially hypokalaemia.
4. Acidosis.
5. Coronary artery disease.
6. Thyrotoxicosis.

Management

1. Correct underlying cause if possible.
2. Connect ECG monitor in order to distinguish supraventricular from ventricular tachycardia.

Supraventricular tachycardia is characterised by normal QRS complexes. P waves may be abnormal or obscured by the T wave of the preceding complex (Figure 4.4). If there is hypotension, synchronised cardioversion should be used without delay, otherwise the following should be considered:

1. Increasing vagal tone by carotid sinus massage, Valsalva manoeuvre or pressure on the eyeball.
2. Adenosine in boluses of 3 mg, 6 mg and 12 mg.

3. Verapamil 5–10 mg i.v. Reduced doses should be used for patients receiving β-blockers.
4. Amiodorone 300 mg slowly.

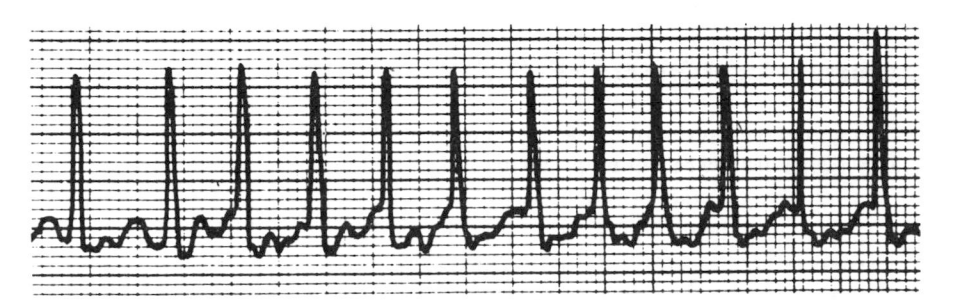

Figure 4.4 Supraventricular tachycardia

Ventricular tachycardia is characterised by wide and abnormal QRS complexes and absence of P waves (Figure 4.5). Treatment as listed below should be instituted without delay, as ventricular fibrillation may follow:

1. Intravenous lignocaine (lidocaine) 1 mg/kg. If a ventricular tachycardia returns or there are frequent ventricular ectopic beats, a lignocaine infusion may be needed.
2. Amiodorone 300 mg slowly.
3. Cardioversion.

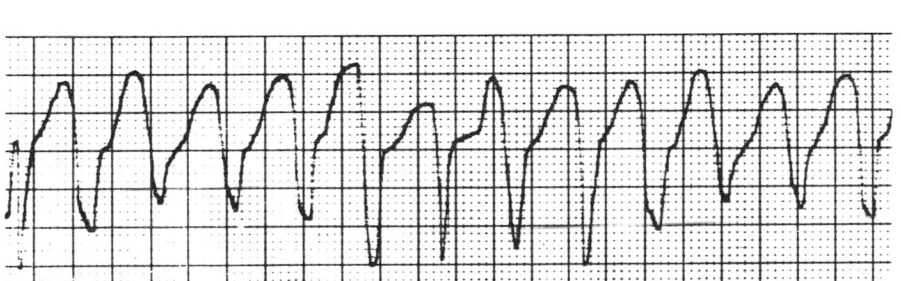

Figure 4.5 Ventricular tachycardia

Dysrhythmias

An irregular pulse in the immediate post-operative period is not an uncommon finding, especially in children.

If the colour is good with the peripheral circulation satisfactory and the blood pressure maintained, no immediate treatment is required. The irregularity is probably due to residual effects of inhalational agents sensitising the myocardium to catecholamines and will pass off as the anaesthetic is eliminated.

If the irregularity persists or is accompanied by hypotension or poor peripheral perfusion, its nature should be established by ECG monitoring.

Although any type of dysrhythmia can occur post-operatively, premature atrial and ventricular contractions and atrial fibrillation are most commonly seen.

Premature Atrial Contractions (PACs)

A premature P wave is followed by a normal QRS complex (Figure 4.6). This dysrhythmia usually causes no problems and no treatment is required.

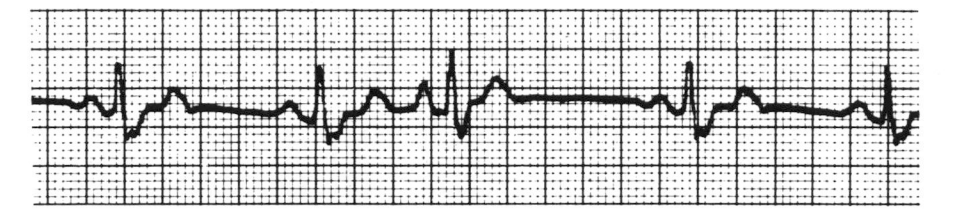

Figure 4.6 Premature atrial contractions

Premature Ventricular Contractions (PVCs)

There is no P wave before a premature QRS complex. The complex is abnormally wide, notched or large and followed by a compensatory pause (Figure 4.7). If premature contractions follow each normal contraction, the term *pulsus bigeminus* is used.

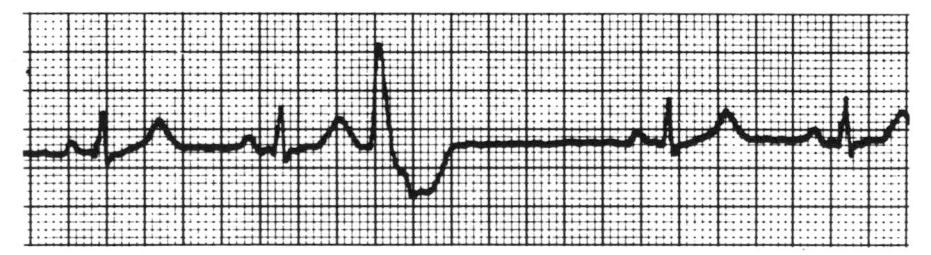

Figure 4.7 Premature ventricular contractions

Causes

1. Hypoxia.
2. Hypercarbia.
3. Acidosis.
4. Hypokalaemia.
5. Digitalis overdose.

6. Excessive circulating catecholamines.
7. Hyperthyroidism.

Management

If the premature beats are infrequent and there is no accompanying hypotension, no treatment is required. If, however, they occur frequently (i.e. more than 5/min), the underlying cause should be sought and corrected, since it may lead to ventricular tachycardia or ventricular fibrillation.

Treatment is by intravenous lignocaine (lidocaine) in a bolus of 1 mg/kg followed by an intravenous infusion at a rate of 1–4 mg/min. Alternatively, a β-blocker such as propranolol or esmolol may be given.

Atrial Fibrillation

P waves are absent and QRS complexes occur irregularly (Figure 4.8). Usually occurs as a result of a long-standing condition, e.g. mitral stenosis or coronary artery disease.

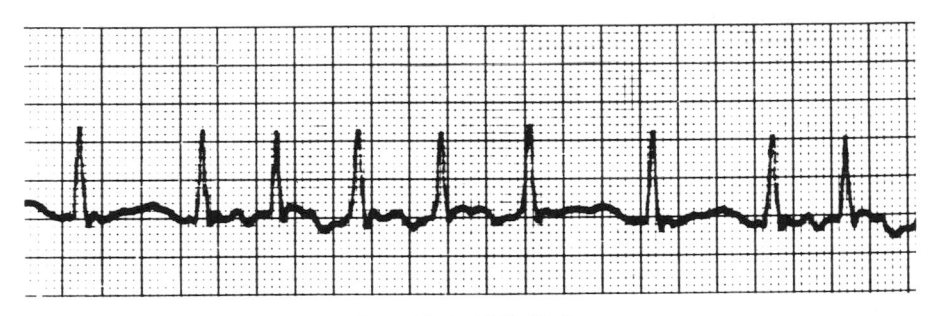

Figure 4.8 Atrial fibrillation

Management

No treatment is required unless the ventricular response is rapid and the pulse rate exceeds 120/minute, or there are accompanying signs of heart failure or hypotension. The following should then be considered:

1. Cardioversion, using a synchronised D.C. shock of 50 J. If this is unsuccessful repeated attempts can be made with an increasing intensity up to 200 J.
2. Digitalisation. This should not precede cardioversion, as the latter may precipitate a cardiac arrest in the digitalised patient.

Many patients with atrial fibrillation are already digitalised prior to surgery so that neither cardioversion nor further digitalisation is appropriate. In this case a slow intravenous injection of disopyramide over 5 min to a total of 2 mg/kg, or until the ventricular rate drops, may be successful.

Cardiac Arrest

Cardiac arrest occurring in the recovery room should be treated vigorously as it has every prospect of success because:

1. The precipitating cause is usually reversible, e.g. hypoxia, electrolyte imbalance, hypovolaemia.
2. The patient is under continuous observation and there may be some advance warning, e.g. hypotension, cyanosis, bradycardia.
3. Resuscitation equipment and trained staff are instantly available.

The diagnosis is made when there is:

1. Loss of consciousness.
2. No breathing.
3. No pulse palpable in a major artery, e.g. in the carotid or femoral.

Examining the pupils, listening for heart sounds or connecting an ECG monitor are unnecessary at this stage. If no major pulse is palpable, cardiopulmonary resuscitation must be commenced without delay.

Initial Management

1. Call for help.
2. Establish a clear airway.
3. Commence artificial ventilation with oxygen using a bag and mask or Ambu bag. If a clear airway is difficult to establish, insertion of a laryngeal mask airway (LMA) may be helpful. As soon as possible the trachea should be intubated with a cuffed endotracheal tube. Give two large breaths ensuring that the lungs are seen to inflate.
4. Commence external cardiac massage by giving vigorous downward thrusts on the lower third of the sternum with the palms of the hands at a rate of 60/min. After five compressions of the heart, pause and inflate the lungs. This cycle must be continued until a spontaneous heartbeat is established.
5. Elevate the foot of the bed to improve venous return.
6. Establish an intravenous infusion, if this is not already present, so that all drugs can be given intravenously.
7. Monitor ECG to establish the electrical activity of the heart. If ventricular fibrillation (Figure 4.9) is shown:
   (a) Give a vigorous pre-cordial thump on the lower sternum with the fist.
   (b) Defibrillate the heart using 200 J (Figure 4.10). If no pulse is palpable immediately after the first shock, continue resuscitation (1:5 ventilation to compressions) while the defibrillator is recharged. Give a second shock.
   (c) If defibrillation fails again, continue resuscitation and then give a third shock of 360 J.

(d) If this is unsuccessful, give intravenous adrenaline 1 mg and continue resuscitation with 10 CPR sequences of 1:5 ventilation to compressions.

(e) Give three further shocks at 360 J and repeat adrenaline 1 mg followed by 10 CPR sequences.

(f) Repeat this cycle three times.

(g) If this fails to establish a normal rhythm give lignocaine 100 mg (10 ml of 1% solution or 5 ml of 2% solution).

(h) If successful, give sodium bicarbonate 50 ml of 8.4% solution.

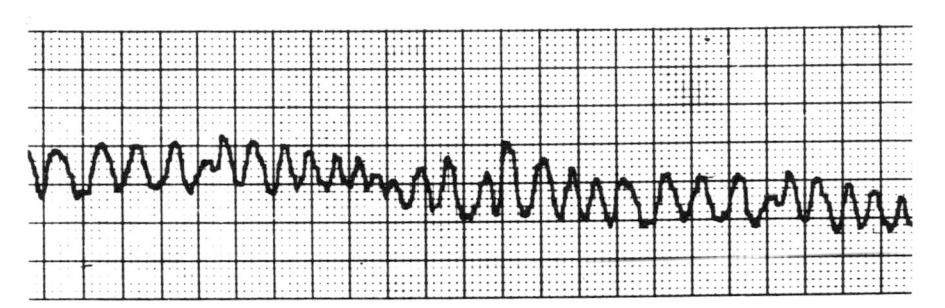

Figure 4.9 Ventricular fibrillation

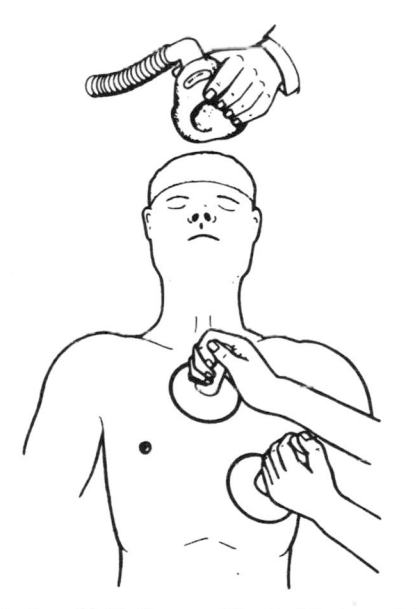

Figure 4.10 Application of defibrillator paddles. Assistants must stand well clear

Ventilation and external cardiac massage should only be interrupted when a D.C. shock is about to be administered.

In refractory ventricular fibrillation, bretylium 400 mg may be tried. It has a slow onset, so resuscitation should be continued even if it initially appears to be ineffective.

8. If, instead of ventricular fibrillation, the monitor shows asystole, ventilation and external cardiac massage should be performed as above and the following administered:
   (a) Two shocks of 200 J and one of 360 J.
   (b) Adrenaline 1 mg intravenously.
   (c) 10 CPR sequences of 1:5 ventilation to compression.
   (d) Atropine 3 mg (once only).
   (e) Repeat steps (b) and (c).

If they fail to produce ventricular fibrillation or a rhythm with a cardiac output, transvenous or oesophageal pacing should be considered.

9. There is a third mechanism of cardiac arrest – electromechanical dissociation. There may be normal or near-normal electrical activity shown on the monitor but it is not accompanied by any useful cardiac output. It has a poor prognosis.
   (a) Consider and exclude mechanical causes such as cardiac tamponade or tension pneumothorax.
   (b) Give adrenaline 1 mg followed by 10 CPR sequences.
   (c) Repeat (b) as required.

If this is unsuccessful consider pressor agents, calcium chloride (10 ml of 10% solution), sodium bicarbonate (50 ml of 8.4% solution) or adrenaline (5 mg).

If there is difficulty inserting an intravenous cannula in a collapsed patient, drugs can be given via the endotracheal tube. Absorption is rapid from the bronchial mucosa. Twice or three times the intravenous dose is usually given. Intracardiac injections are hazardous, offer few advantages and are best avoided.

Once a spontaneous heartbeat has been re-established and any precipitating factors corrected, the patient should be transferred to an intensive-care unit so that intensive monitoring and further treatment can be given:

1. Ensure breathing is adequate. Consider a period of artificial ventilation. If a pneumothorax is suspected, insert a chest drain.
2. Estimate arterial blood gases – further bicarbonate may be necessary.
3. Estimate serum potassium.
4. Obtain a chest X-ray.
5. Measure the arterial blood pressure.
6. Insert a urinary catheter and monitor the urine output.
7. Insert a nasogastric tube and aspirate the stomach contents.
8. Insert a central venous catheter if indicated.
9. Obtain a 12-lead ECG.
10. Consider high-dose steroids to protect an ischaemic brain.

The treatment of a cardiac arrest is modified for paediatric patients. A summary of the management for both adults and children is given in Figures 4.11 and 4.12 (*overleaf*).

MISCELLANEOUS COMPLICATIONS

Delayed Return of Consciousness

Most patients will have regained consciousness within 15 min of arrival in the recovery room. If unconsciousness persists for longer than 30 min a cause should be sought.

Causes

1. Drugs:
   (a) Relative overdose of drugs:
       (i) Excess administration, e.g. premedication, opiate supplements.
       (ii) Increased sensitivity, e.g. extremes of age, cachectic or hypothyroid patient.
       (iii) Diminished metabolism, e.g. in liver dysfunction, hypothermia, hypothyroidism.
   (b) Drugs with prolonged action, e.g. ketamine, droperidol, lorazepam, repeat doses of barbiturates.
2. Hypoglycaemia.
3. Hypercarbia.
4. Metabolic acidosis.
5. Cerebral damage, which may result from a period of cerebral hypoxia or from a cerebrovascular accident during anaesthesia.
6. Uraemia.

Management

1. Ensure that the airway is clear and that respiration is adequate.
2. Reverse depression with specific antagonists if the cause is known. In the case of opiates, naloxone up to 0.4 mg can be given, carefully titrating the dose according to the patient's response. Once the desired effect has been produced, further doses should be avoided as these will reverse the analgesic effect. Depression due to benzodiazepines can be reversed by flumazenil 300–600 mcg.
3. Check blood sugar. Treat hypoglycaemia with 50 ml of 50% glucose intravenously.
4. Check blood gases to exclude hypercarbia or metabolic acidosis. Treat with assisted ventilation or intravenous sodium bicarbonate, as appropriate.
5. Consider flumazenil if benzodiazepines have been given.
6. Make a thorough examination of the central nervous system, taking a special

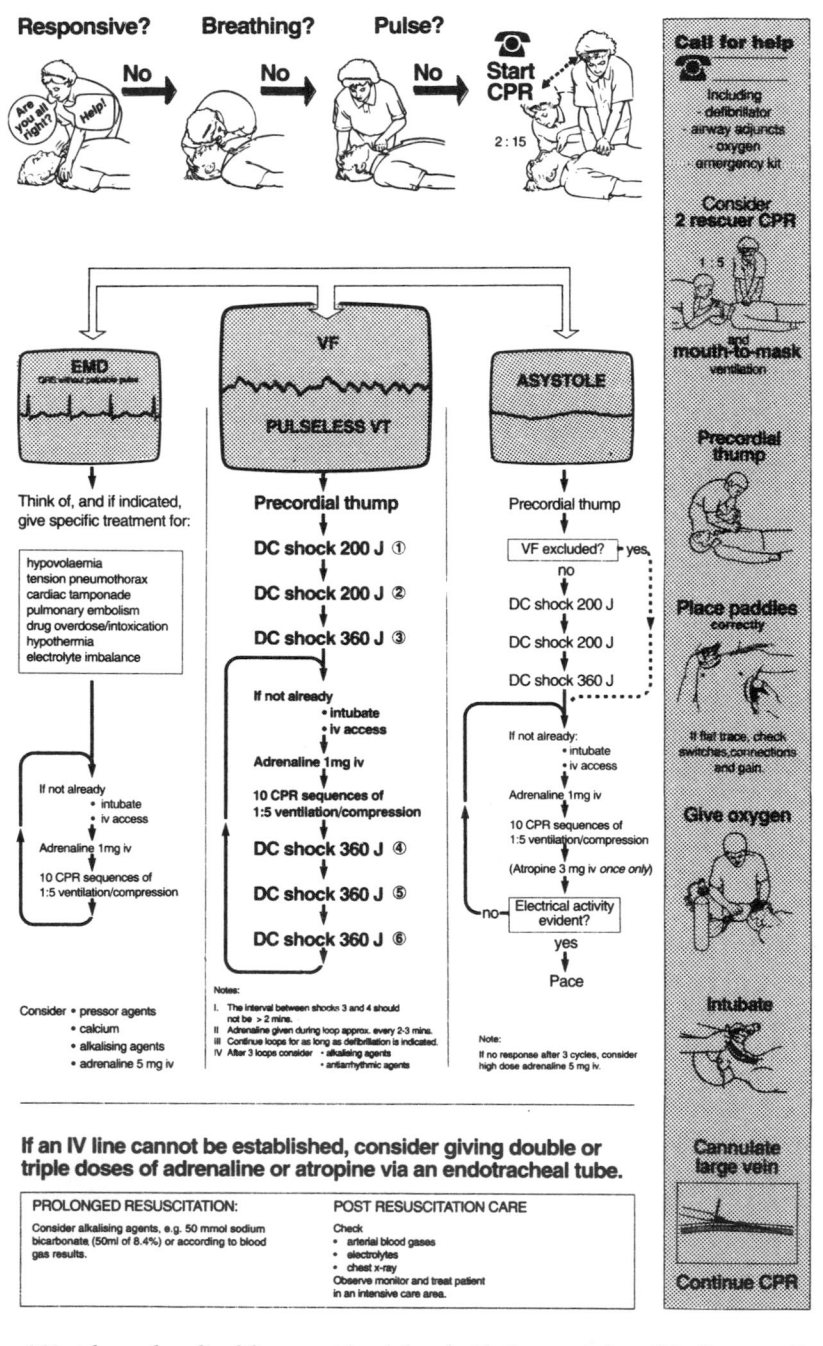

Figure 4.11 Advanced cardiac life support (reproduced with the permission of the European Resuscitation Council)

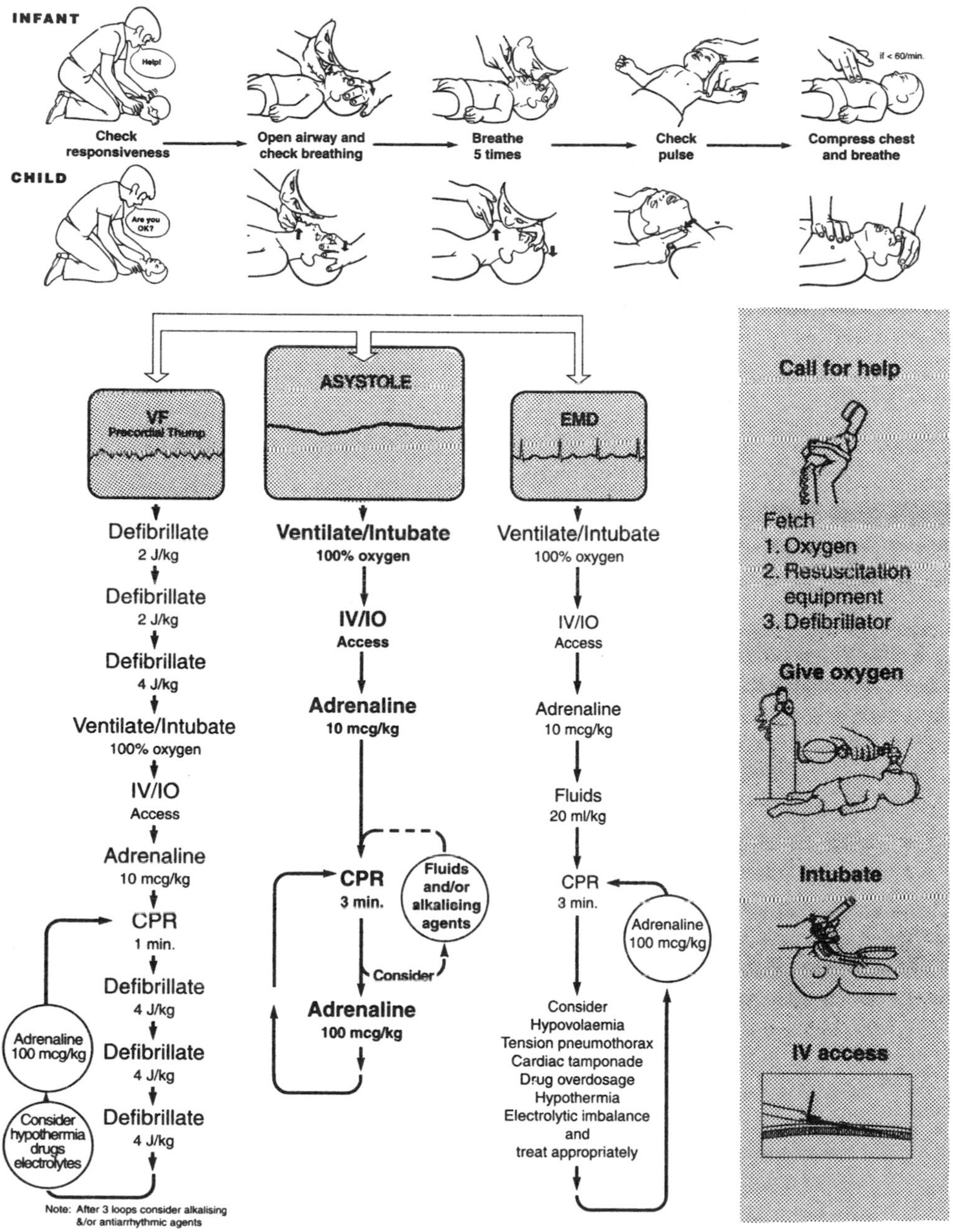

Figure 4.12 Paediatric advanced life support (reproduced with the permission of the European Resuscitation Council)

note of localising signs, and record the findings as a baseline for future reference.

7. If there is still no response after 2–3h and the obvious causes have been treated, the patient should be transferred to an intensive-care unit for subsequent management.

Restlessness, Excitement and Delirium

The immediate post-operative period may be accompanied by various degrees of excitement ranging from mild restlessness to violent uncontrolled movement.

Causes

1. Airway obstruction, especially caused by nasal packs (see page 122).
2. Anxiety.
3. Pain.
4. Full bladder.
5. Inadequate reversal of muscle relaxants.
6. Cerebral hypoxia.
7. Drugs. Elderly patients in particular can be extremely sensitive to drugs used in premedication, e.g. hyoscine, phenothiazines and barbiturates, and to ketamine.
8. Middle-ear surgery. Restlessness is frequent following this type of surgery, possibly due to a temporary disturbance of the labyrinthine mechanism.
9. Raised intracranial pressure.
10. Hyperthyroidism.
11. Psychological distress, e.g. following termination of pregnancy.

Management

1. *Reassurance.* Anxious patients finding themselves in unfamiliar surroundings may become restless. They will frequently settle with gentle handling and sympathetic reassurance.
2. *Restraint.* Care must be taken to prevent the more vigorous patients from injuring themselves. Cot sides should be raised. If it is necessary for patients to be restrained, minimal force should be used.
3. *Analgesics.* Administration should be intravenous, as required to relieve pain. Many patients will be unable to complain of pain in the immediate post-operative period. However, in the absence of other obvious causes, restlessness, especially if accompanied by tachycardia and hypertension, will usually respond to analgesic therapy.

4. *Give oxygen by face mask.*
5. *Ensure adequate reversal of relaxants,* giving further atropine and neo-stigmine if required. If ventilation remains inadequate, intubation and assisted ventilation may be needed.
6. *Catheterise the bladder* if it is distended.
7. Following trauma or neurosurgery, raised intracranial pressure must always be considered, especially if the restlessness is accompanied by hypertension and bradycardia. If this is the case, a *neurological observation chart* should be commenced at once and further advice sought.

Nausea and Vomiting

With improvements in anaesthetic drugs and techniques over the years, the incidence of post-operative vomiting has undoubtedly decreased. However, as one can never be absolutely certain that the stomach is empty even in fasted patients, recovery staff must be alert to the possibility of vomiting.

Causes

Various individual factors contribute to the incidence of post-operative vomiting. The results of numerous studies have shown it to be more frequent:

1. In those prone to motion sickness.
2. In females rather than males.
3. Following the use of ether.
4. With increasing duration of anaesthesia.
5. Following the use of opiates. The effect is exacerbated with early mobilisation and reduced with the concurrent use of atropine, hyoscine or anti-histamines.
6. Following episodes of hypoxia or hypotension.
7. Following intra-abdominal surgery.
8. In the presence of severe pain.
9. After middle ear surgery.
10. Following the use of nitrous oxide.

Management

Because of the danger of respiratory obstruction or aspiration resulting from vomiting, the recovery patient should be nursed on a tipping trolley and with suction apparatus to hand. Unless contraindicated (e.g. because of orthopaedic traction), patients should normally be on their sides so as to enable vomited material to be cleared from the pharynx by gravity. In the event of vomiting:

1. Tip the head down.

2. Suck out the pharynx.
3. Turn the patient on to his side, if he is not already in this position (normally on the left side in case subsequent laryngoscopy is required). This requires the help of an assistant.
4. If respiratory obstruction persists, clear the pharynx under direct vision using a laryngoscope.
5. Give oxygen by face mask.

For treatment of aspiration of gastric contents, see page 78.

When vomiting or nausea persists for more than a brief period and pain can be excluded as a cause, anti-emetics such as prochlorperazine, metoclopramide or droperidol may be given intravenously or intramuscularly. In resistant cases the 5-HT$_3$ antagonist ondansetron has been shown to be effective. The routine use of anti-emetics, however, is not recommended since persistent vomiting is not a problem in the majority of patients. Prophylactic anti-emetics are given:

1. Where vomiting is particularly undesirable, such as following a perforating eye injury, where it may cause a rise in intra-ocular pressure, or when the jaws have been wired together and suction is difficult.
2. If there is a history of post-operative vomiting.

Following anti-emetic therapy, extra-pyramidal effects (e.g. muscle rigidity, restlessness, oculogyric crisis) have sometimes occurred, particularly after repeated doses of long-acting agents. These are very frightening to the patient and can be treated with anti-Parkinson-type drugs such as benzhexol or procyclidine.

Shivering

Shivering is frequently seen during recovery from general anaesthesia and may be so severe as to resemble grand mal epilepsy.

Causes

1. *Inhalational anaesthetic agents.* Shivering is commonest after the use of halothane but may follow other agents. The exact mechanism is unclear, although it has been shown to be unrelated to temperature change.
2. *Blood transfusion reactions* (page 103).
3. *Hypothermia* (page 100).
4. *Epidural anaesthesia.*

Management

Although shivering is usually transient and does not often pose a problem, the following measures can be taken:

1. *Administration of oxygen* to increase F_iO_2. Shivering increases metabolic rate and so causes excess oxygen demand. Demand may exceed supply unless additional oxygen is administered.
2. *Rewarm the patient* if there is significant hypothermia (page 100).

Convulsions

Causes

1. *Cerebral irritation* owing to:
   (a) Trauma.
   (b) Neurosurgery.
   (c) A hypoxic episode.
   (d) Presence of intracranial mass.
2. *Febrile convulsions*. The combination of:
   (a) Pre-operative pyrexia.
   (b) Dehydration.
   (c) Atropine premedication, which reduces sweating.
   (d) Inhalational anaesthetics, which may interfere with the heat-regulating centre (especially diethyl ether).
   (e) Excessive coverings reducing heat loss especially in children.
3. *Epilepsy*, particularly if anticonvulsant drugs have been omitted prior to surgery.
4. *Drugs:*
   (a) Local anaesthetics – convulsions may result if the total quantity injected is excessive or if there has been an inadvertent intravascular injection. Special care is required when releasing a tourniquet following a Bier's block and when topping up an epidural in the recovery room in case the tip of the catheter has migrated into a vein.
   (b) Diethyl ether, especially when accompanied by dehydration or fever.
   (c) Enflurane, especially in high concentrations with hyperventilation.
   (d) Methohexitone (methohexital).
5. *Eclampsia.* Preventative measures against convulsions must be continued into the post-operative period (page 118).
6. *Hypoglycaemia.*
7. *Dilutional hyponatraemia* (page 135).
8. *Uraemia.*

Management

Regardless of the cause, oxygen is administered and convulsions terminated as rapidly as possible because of the dangers posed by an uncontrolled airway and excessive oxygen demand. Thiopentone (thiopental), midazolam, pheno-barbitone (phenobarbital) and sodium valproate (valproic acid) are suitable drugs for this purpose. In extreme cases, muscle relaxants, such as suxa-methonium (succinylcholine), intubation and artificial respiration may be needed. Once the convulsions have been controlled, attempts should be made to determine the underlying cause and to correct it.

Hypothermia

Agents used during general anaesthesia may depress the heat-regulating centre in the hypothalamus, causing vasodilation or impaired shivering. Consequently some fall in temperature is not uncommon post-operatively, but with the use of thermostatically controlled operating theatres, this is seldom severe except at the extremes of age.

Causes

1. Prolonged bowel exposure.
2. Prolonged surgery in infants (because of their greater tendency to lose heat, see page 140).
3. Intravenous infusions of large volumes of cold solutions or blood.
4. Following deliberate hypothermia employed during cardiac or neurosurgery.
5. Hypothyroidism.
6. Bladder irrigation with cold fluids.

   Hypothermia may lead to:

1. Myocardial depression or irritability.
2. Metabolic acidosis.
3. Altered response to neuromuscular blocking agents.
4. Poor respiratory effort and hypoxia, particularly in children.

Management

1. Prevent further heat loss by supplying extra warmed blankets or wrapping the patient in an aluminium-foil space blanket. Rewarming can be achieved rapidly by using a specially designed hot-air warming blanket, e.g. the "Warm Touch" blanket.
2. Give intravenous fluids through a warming coil.
3. In the case of infants, the use of a warmed incubator or overhead heater is recommended.
4. Monitor temperature. This should be done continuously if possible or at frequent intervals. The core temperature is a more valuable guide than skin

temperature and this can be measured conveniently by a tympanic membrane thermometer. Alternatively, a nasopharyngeal, oesophageal or rectal probe can be used. A low-reading thermometer may be necessary in extreme cases.

5. Keep the patient in the recovery unit until his temperature has risen above 35°C.

6. In neonates, hypothermia can interfere with respiratory effort. If this occurs intubation and assisted ventilation may be required until normothermia has been achieved.

Hyperthermia

A moderate rise in temperature (e.g. up to 39°C) unaccompanied by other signs or symptoms does not in itself constitute a problem. However, the origin should be sought since it may require treatment in the recovery room.

Causes

1. *Infection.* This may have been present before surgery or may first become apparent immediately afterwards, especially following bowel or urological surgery.

2. *Impaired heat loss.* The combination of pre-operative pyrexia, atropine (which reduces sweating), a high ambient temperature and the use of agents which interfere with the heat-regulating centre (especially diethyl ether) can cause hyperthermia, particularly in children.

3. *Pyrogens* introduced during blood transfusion.

4. *Malignant hyperpyrexia* (see overleaf).

Management

1. Where infection is considered likely, appropriate antibiotic therapy should be commenced intravenously. If blood culture is contemplated, it should precede the administration of antibiotics.

2. If hyperthermia follows blood transfusion this should be stopped immediately and a sample of the transfused blood saved for analysis (page 108).

3. Severe hyperpyrexia (> 39°C), especially in children, will result in increased oxygen consumption and carbon dioxide production with metabolic and respiratory acidosis, causing increased demands on cardiac and respiratory function. This may result in cerebral hypoxia and convulsions, and should be treated vigorously by:
   (a) Active cooling with tepid sponging, ice and fans.
   (b) Oxygen therapy.
   (c) Intravenous midazolam as required to control convulsions.

Malignant Hyperthermia

This is a rare condition of unknown aetiology characterised by a rise in temperature of up to 1°C every 15 min which can be rapidly fatal unless treated immediately. It is often triggered by anaesthesia and especially by the use of suxamethonium (succinylcholine) or halothane, although other anaesthetic agents and relaxants have been implicated. Evidence suggests that there is a hereditary defect in the calcium-storing membrane of the skeletal and cardiac muscle cells so that calcium is released into the cytoplasm with the production of heat.

The temperature rise may immediately follow the triggering mechanism or there may be an interval of 30–45 min, so that it may not become obvious until the patient has reached the recovery room.

Clinical Features

1. Extreme pyrexia.
2. Cyanosis.
3. Tachycardia and tachypnoea.
4. Metabolic and respiratory acidosis.
5. Hyperkalaemia.
6. Muscle rigidity (in 60% of patients).
7. Coagulopathy.

Management

1. Hyperventilation with 100% oxygen.
2. Vigorous cooling with ice and fans.
3. Sodium bicarbonate to correct acidosis (monitoring of blood gases will be required).
4. Intravenous dextrose 50 ml of 50% and 10 units of soluble insulin to reduce hyperkalaemia.
5. Intravenous dantrolene 1 mg/kg every 5 min (up to 10 mg/kg may be required). Dantrolene inhibits the release of calcium into the muscle cell.
6. Intravenous frusemide (furosemide) or mannitol to increase urinary output and prevent casts of myoglobin from blocking the renal tubules.

Because of the rapidity of onset and the urgency of treatment, a malignant hyperthermia pack with all the necessary drugs should be readily available in the recovery room.

Following an episode of malignant hyperpyrexia this must be carefully recorded in the patient's notes and the family practitioner should be notified so that other members of the family can be screened for this abnormality.

Blood Transfusion Reactions

Blood transfusion may be in progress when patients are admitted to the recovery room, or alternatively may become necessary during the immediate post-operative period. In either event, recovery staff must be alert for transfusion reactions which may be febrile, allergic or haemolytic. As patients are covered with drapes during surgery, skin reactions may only become obvious when these are removed at the end of the procedure.

Febrile Reactions

Febrile reactions occur in 1–2% of transfusions and are generally caused by anti-leucocyte antibodies in the transfused blood. They are relatively slow in onset, the usual time from the start of transfusion being 2–4 h. Reactions may be more severe when blood is being transfused rapidly.

1. *Mild febrile reactions:* Temperature below 39°C, no other symptoms or signs.
   (a) Slow transfusion rate.
   (b) Administer antipyretics, e.g. paracetamol (acetaminophen).
2. *Severe febrile reactions:* Temperature above 39°C, accompanied by rigors.
   (a) Stop transfusion.
   (b) Actively cool the patient with tepid sponging and fans.
   Bacterial contamination of transfused blood may initially present in this way. If this is suspected or there are accompanying signs of cardiovascular collapse:
   (a) Give a broad-spectrum antibiotic.
   (b) Support the circulation by intravenous infusion.
   (c) Take appropriate blood samples and return the unit of blood and any previous units to the blood bank for bacteriological examination and serological testing.

Allergic Reactions

1. *Mild:* Itching, rash.
   (a) Continue transfusion.
   (b) Administer antihistamines, e.g. chlorpheniramine 10 mg i.m.
2. *Severe:* Oedema, bronchospasm, hypotension.
   (a) Stop transfusion.
   (b) Support circulation by intravenous infusion.
   (c) Administer hydrocortisone 100 mg i.v.
   (d) Consider adrenaline (epinephrine) 1 mg (1 ml 1:1000 solution) i.v.

Haemolytic Reactions

Haemolytic reactions are caused by incompatible blood transfusion. Haemolysed red cells release free haemoglobin which can cause renal damage. Reactions are characterised by:

1. Localised pain.
2. Loin or retrosternal pain. $\Big\}$ These signs are masked by unconsciousness
3. Flushing.
4. Pyrexia.
5. Dyspnoea.
6. Cardiovascular collapse.
7. Oliguria.
8. Haematuria.

The picture may be complicated in 50% of patients by the development of disseminated intravascular coagulation. If this occurs:

1. Stop transfusion and take down the giving set.
2. Support circulation by intravenous infusion.
3. Give intravenous hydrocortisone 1 g.
4. Send the unit of blood and any previously used packs, together with a clotted sample of blood and anticoagulated samples, for platelet count, clotting studies and examination for free Hb (page 108).
5. Catheterise the bladder and monitor urine output. Send sample of urine for examination for Hb and urobilinogen.
6. Stimulate urine production with frusemide (furosemide) or mannitol.
7. Alkalinise urine with i.v. sodium bicarbonate to increase solubility of free Hb.

Problems Associated with Massive Blood Transfusion

In addition to the normal hazards of any blood transfusion, whenever large volumes of blood have to be transfused rapidly (e.g. 500 ml every 5 min for 30 min), further problems may be anticipated as a result of changes in the stored blood.

Hypothermia

Since blood is normally stored at 4°C, the rapid infusion of cold blood will reduce body temperature and lead to:

1. Dysrhythmias and, in extreme cases, cardiac arrest.
2. A shift of the oxygen dissociation curve to the left with impairment of oxygen release in the tissues.

To eliminate these complications, large transfusions of blood should first pass through a blood warmer so that when it is transfused it is at body temperature.

Acidosis

Stored blood becomes progressively more acidotic and may have a pH of below 7.0. This is partly due to the presence of citrate in the anticoagulant and partly due to continuing anaerobic metabolism with lactic acid production. Since the shocked patient may already be acidotic, the resulting pH may become so low that it interferes with myocardial function and the reversal of muscle relaxants. This can be corrected by giving sodium bicarbonate intravenously, titrating the amount according to serial acid–base determinations. Bicarbonate should not, however, be given routinely as a metabolic alkalosis may result and further impair myocardial function.

Citrate Intoxication

Ionised calcium in stored blood is reduced by binding the citrate which is used as an anticoagulant. Under normal circumstances, the body has sufficient stores of calcium in the skeleton to compensate for this. However, following a massive transfusion or when citrate metabolism is impaired by liver disease, hypocalcaemia may result. This causes myocardial depression and hypotension. On the ECG, the ST segment is prolonged.

The treatment is to give 10 ml of 10% calcium gluconate slowly until the hypotension and ECG abnormalities are corrected.

Hyperkalaemia

Potassium diffuses from red cells during storage at a rate approaching 1 mmol per day so that at the end of 28 days' storage, blood may contain up to 30 mmol/l. This may lead to significant hyperkalaemia (especially if renal function is impaired) with high peaked T waves on ECG and cardiac irritability. These effects can be countered by giving calcium gluconate, as described above. Alternatively, as insulin causes potassium to move intracellularly, 10 units of soluble insulin and 50 ml 50% dextrose can be given.

Micro-emboli

Stored blood contains microaggregates consisting of cell remnants and threads of fibrin ranging in diameter from 20 to 200 μm. Following transfusion these are filtered by the microcirculation of the lungs and may lead to the development of adult respiratory distress syndrome (ARDS). This effect can be minimised by passing blood through a microfilter of pore size 20–40 μm and this is recommended by some workers for large transfusions, especially when old blood is used. The resulting increased resistance to the blood transfusion can be overcome by using a pressure bag to maintain flow.

Failure of Coagulation (*see also* the next section)

Stored blood rapidly becomes deficient in clotting factors (especially V, VII and VIII) and platelets, so that following a massive transfusion, their levels may become significantly reduced. These deficiencies can normally be made good with fresh frozen plasma (one unit for every five units of blood) and platelet concentrate (one unit for every ten units of blood). Coagulation studies will be required if bleeding persists despite this regimen.

Failure of Coagulation

Persistent bleeding in the immediate post-operative period may be due to defective coagulation. Damage to blood vessels results in an accumulation of platelets around which a fibrin clot is formed. A variety of clotting factors must be present in the blood to allow the conversion of fibrinogen into the fibrin filaments:

I	Fibrinogen
II	Prothrombin
III	Thromboplastin
IV	Calcium
V	Pro-accelerin
VI	Not allocated
VII	Pro-convertin
VIII	Anti-haemophilic factor
IX	Christmas factor
X	Stuart-Power factor
XI	Plasma thromboplastin antecedent
XII	Hageman factor
XIII	Fibrin stabilising factor

The fibrin clot is eventually lysed by plasmin, which is formed by conversion of the inactive plasminogen.

Causes

1. *Congenital deficiency of clotting factors.* Normally a single factor is deficient, e.g. haemophilia A (factor VIII) or Christmas disease (factor IX). This is usually recognised prior to surgery and the deficient factor is replaced pre- and post-operatively. This requires frequent assays of the appropriate factor. Formerly, some preparations of these factors were contaminated with the AIDS virus and many haemophiliacs were infected. The preparations currently used carry no risk.
2. *Massive blood transfusion.* Stored blood rapidly becomes deficient in clotting factors (especially V, VII and VIII) and subsequently in platelets. In addition,

calcium is bound by the citrate anticoagulant and the resulting hypocalcaemia may contribute to deficient coagulation.

3. *Anticoagulants:*

   (a) *Heparin* acts at several sites in the coagulation process. It is frequently
   given intravenously during cardiovascular surgery and may be reversed
   by protamine sulphate. Care must be taken with protamine treatment
   since in excess amounts it may also act as an anticoagulant.

   (b) *Coumarin-type drugs*, e.g. warfarin sodium. These inhibit the vitamin K-
   dependent carboxylation of clotting factors II, VII, IX and X in the liver.
   Rapid reversal cannot therefore be achieved by simply giving intravenous vitamin K preparations such as phytomenadione (phytonadione),
   as fresh clotting factors have to be synthesised in the liver. If rapid reversal of anticoagulation is required, fresh frozen plasma should be
   given.

4. *Liver disease.* Most clotting factors are synthesised in the liver and may be
   deficient in severe liver dysfunction.

5. *Vitamin K deficiency.* Vitamin K absorption is impaired in obstructive
   jaundice and following pre-operative bowel sterilisation with antibiotics.

6. *Disseminated intravascular coagulation (DIC).* In the following clinical states
   there is massive deposition of fibrin throughout the microcirculation,
   resulting in the consumption of clotting factors and platelets with consequent
   bleeding:

   (a) Prolonged shock with tissue hypoxia.

   (b) Extensive tissue damage, e.g. trauma, burns, prolonged surgery.

   (c) Infection, e.g. acute viral infection, septicaemia.

   (d) Obstetric emergencies, e.g. amniotic fluid embolism, intra-uterine death,
   abruptio placentae, toxaemia.

   (e) Acute haemolysis, e.g. mismatched transfusion.

   (f) Following prostatectomy.

   (g) Extracorporeal circulation.

   Extensive fibrinolysis follows, with the liberation of fibrin degradation
   products and thence further bleeding. The condition is therefore characterised by clotting and bleeding occurring simultaneously.

7. *Thrombocytopaenia* (platelet deficiency). Platelets are not only required to
   initiate haemostasis by plugging damaged blood vessels but are also essential
   in the coagulation process. If the platelet count falls below 50×10^9/litre, a
   failure of coagulation may occur.

   Causes of thrombocytopaenia seen post-operatively:

   (a) *Dilution of platelets.* Transfusion of stored blood which is deficient in
   platelets leads to a reduction in circulating platelet count. This reduction
   is more than can be accounted for by dilution alone. Significant reduction in platelet count is often observed after the rapid transfusion of six
   or more units of stored blood.

(b) *Depressed platelet formation,* e.g. as seen in patients with leukaemia, cancer, uraemia and during chemotherapy.

(c) *Excessive utilisation of platelets,* e.g. in disseminated intravascular coagulation.

(d) *Idiopathic thrombocytopaenia.* A rare condition of unknown aetiology seen mainly in young adults and characterised by purpura and petechiae.

(e) *Excessive destruction of platelets,* e.g. in hypersplenism.

Management

To determine the cause of a failure of coagulation will require a series of laboratory tests:

1. *Platelet count* (EDTA bottle). Normal values 150×10^9/litre to 400×10^9/litre. Bleeding is unusual if the value is above 50×10^9/litre.

2. *Prothrombin time* (sodium citrate bottle). Normal value, approximately 12 s. Therapeutic ratio is 2–4 times the normal value. Prolonged in deficiency of factors II, V, VIII and X, e.g. as seen in liver disease, vitamin K deficiency, anticoagulant therapy and DIC.

3. *Activated partial thromboplastin time* (APTT) (sodium citrate bottle); also kaolin cephalin clotting time (KCCT). Normal values, 25–40 s. Prolonged in deficiency factors II, V, VIII, X, XI and XII, e.g. as seen in anticoagulant therapy, haemophilia A, Christmas disease.

4. *Fibrin degradation products* (FDPs) (bottle with soya bean trypsin inhibitor). Normal values $< 10 \, \mu g$/ml. Raised in DIC. (Smaller rises are found following major surgery, trauma, deep vein thrombosis and pulmonary embolism.)

5. *D. dymers.* This is an alternative investigation for DIC. It has the advantage that it can be estimated from a standard citrate bottle. Normal values $< 0.5 \, \mu g$/ml.

6. *Fibrinogen level* (sodium citrate bottle). In this test the plasma is diluted to give the titre, i.e. the greater the fibrinogen content the more the dilution. Normal values > 1:64; low values < 1:64. The test may be modified to detect the presence of a circulating inhibitor or fibrinolysins. Fibrinogen is deficient in liver disease, in DIC and after massive blood transfusion.

7. *Thrombin clotting time* (TCT) (sodium citrate bottle). Normal values, 20–30 s. Prolonged when fibrinogen is deficient or abnormal and in the presence of inhibitory substances, e.g. FDPs, heparin.

The above tests are not, however, necessary for rational therapy to be given; the immediate history will usually supply sufficient information for this purpose.

1. *Following massive transfusion of stored blood* it can be predicted that clotting factors, platelets and available calcium will be reduced. This can be corrected by the administration of:

(a) Fresh frozen plasma. This contains all the clotting factors and can normally be made available within 20 min. Adequate levels can be maintained by giving one unit of fresh frozen plasma for every five units of blood.

(b) Platelet concentrate. This has to be prepared at a transfusion centre from freshly donated blood. As it deteriorates rapidly it should be used without delay. The standard type of blood filter should not be used for the infusion of platelets. A specially designated filter is usually supplied with platelets.

(c) Intravenous calcium gluconate 10%. Increments of 10 ml may be needed for every litre of blood transfused rapidly. This is mainly to counter myocardial depression due to hypocalcaemia, which only rarely interferes with coagulation.

2. *Following cardiovascular surgery* persistent heparinisation may require reversal by intravenous protamine sulphate. In calculating dosage, allowance should be made for the metabolism of heparin. Minimally effective amounts should be used since excess protamine itself interferes with coagulation.

If these simple measures do not correct the situation and the clinical picture suggests the possibility of disseminated intravascular coagulation, further action is urgently required:

1. *Consult a haematologist.* It is wise to enlist the help of an experienced haematologist at an early stage since inappropriate therapy will not only waste valuable time but also make subsequent management more difficult.

2. *Draw blood for coagulation tests.* As the coagulation profile may be constantly changing, it is important that all the blood required for the various tests is taken at the same time.

3. *Continue to replace blood* with the addition of fresh frozen plasma, platelets and calcium as required to prevent further deficiencies.

In the event of DIC being diagnosed, subsequent treatment will be aimed at:

1. Removal of precipitating stimulus if possible, e.g. evacuation of uterine contents.

2. Replacement of coagulation factors and, possibly:

3. Heparinisation – despite persistent bleeding this may be necessary to prevent continued intravascular coagulation with consumption of clotting factors.

Oliguria

Causes

Inadequate urine output (less than 0.5 ml/(kg h)) may be due to the following causes:

1. *Pre-renal.* Inadequate renal perfusion owing to hypovolaemia or hypotension,

e.g. systolic readings of below 60 mmHg.

2. *Renal damage* due to:
    (a) Sepsis.
    (b) Haemolysis.
    (c) Hypoxaemia.
    (d) Hypotension.
    (e) Antibiotic therapy, e.g. gentamicin.
    (f) Release of myoglobin, e.g. following crush injury, malignant hyperthermia, mismatched transfusion.
3. *Post-renal outflow obstruction* owing to blood clot or kinked urinary catheter.

The urine output is monitored post-operatively in patients at risk of developing acute renal failure. Indications include:

1. Impaired renal or cardiac function pre-operatively.
2. Obstructive jaundice (see page 153).
3. Episodes of hypoxia or hypotension.
4. Cardiac or aortic surgery.
5. Major trauma or severe blood loss.
6. Septicaemia.
7. Extensive burns.
8. Crush injury.
9. Mismatched transfusion.
10. Pancreatitis.
11. Malignant hyperthermia.

Management

1. Exclude mechanical obstruction of urinary catheter caused by clots of blood or kinking. Bladder distension will suggest this. Change catheter if obstruction cannot be cleared.
2. Consider hypotension or hypovolaemia as the most likely causes. Measure the CVP, if necessary.
3. Infuse 250–500 ml of sodium chloride 0.9% intravenously. A subsequent increase in urine output confirms hypovolaemia, which must be corrected.

If these measures are unsuccessful and the urine production remains below 0.5 ml/(kg h), acute renal failure may be imminent.

4. Urinary production may be stimulated by:
    (a) Mannitol 100 ml of 20% over 15 min.
    (b) Frusemide (furosemide) 20–40 mg.
    (c) Low-dose dopamine infusion, i.e. up to 5 µg/(kg min).

If an adequate renal output is not established following these measures, acute renal failure must be assumed to have occurred and the advice of a nephrologist should be sought as soon as possible. While the patient remains in the recovery unit it is important not to overload the circulation.

References and Bibliography

Anderson R, Krohg K (1976). Pain as a major cause of post-operative nausea. Can Anaesth Soc, 23, 366–369.

Asbury AJ (1981). Problems of the immediate post-anaesthesia period. Br J Hosp Med, 25, 159–163.

Bay J, Nunn JF, Prys-Roberts C (1968). Factors influencing arterial PO_2 during recovery from anaesthesia. Br J Anaesth, 40, 398–407.

Bevan DR (1979). Renal function in anaesthesia and surgery. Academic Press, London.

Buckley JJ, Jackson JA (1961). Post-operative cardiac arrhythmias. Anaesthesiol, 22, 723–737.

Calhoun DA, Operail S (1990). Treatment of hypertensive crisis. Cur Con, 323, 1177–1183.

Cullen DJ, Cullen BL (1975). Post-anaesthetic complications. Surg Clin North Am, 55, 987–998.

Darbyshire P (1988). C.V.P. monitoring. Nursing Times, 24(6), 36–38.

Drain CB, Shipley SB (1979). Recovery Room. WB Saunders, Philadelphia.

Evans TR (Ed) (1986). ABC of Resuscitation. BMJ publications, London.

Farman JV (1978). The work of the recovery room. Br J Hosp Med, 19, 606–616.

Farman JV, Hudson RBS, Andrewes S, Eltringham RJ (1979). Symposium: recovery from anaesthesia. J R Soc Med, 72, 270–280.

Feeley TW (1980). The recovery room. In: Miller RD (Ed), Anaesthesia, Churchill Livingstone, Edinburgh and New York.

Gal TJ, Cooperman LH (1975). Hypertension in the immediate post-operative period. Br J Anaesth, 47, 70–74.

Goldman L. (1995). Cardiac risk in non-cardiac surgery: an update. Anaes Analg, 80, 810–820.

Greenwalt TJ (Ed) (1988). Blood transfusion. American Medical Association, Wisconsin.

Hanson GC, Wright PL (Eds) (1978). The Medical Management of the Critically Ill. Academic Press, London, and Grune and Stratton, New York.

Jones RM, Hantler CB, Knight PR (1981). Use of pentolinium in post-operative hypertension resistant to sodium nitroprusside. Br J Anaesth, 53, 1151–1154.

Marshall BE, Wyche MQ (1972). Hypoxaemia during and after anaesthesia. Anaesthesiol, 37, 178–209.

Seeley HF (1978). The clinical management of the aspiration of gastric contents. J Int Med Res, Suppl I, 63–69.

Smith DC et al (1989). Pulse oximetry in the recovery room. Anaesthesia, 44(4), 345–348.

Stoddart JC (1978). Post-operative respiratory failure: an anaesthetic hazard? Br J Anaesth, 50, 695–700.

Taylor TH, Major E (1993). Hazards and Complications of Anaesthesia. Churchill Livingstone, Edinburgh.

White JC (1982). The relief of post-operative pain. In: Atkinson RS, Hewer CL (Eds), Recent Adv Anaesth Analg, 14, Churchill Livingstone, Edinburgh, pp. 121–139.

Wynne JW, Modell JH (1977). Respiratory aspiration of stomach contents. Ann Intern Med, 87, 466–474.

Chapter 5
RECOVERY IN DIFFERENT BRANCHES OF SURGERY

EMERGENCY SURGERY

Many patients will present for emergency surgery without time for adequate pre-operative preparation. In some cases, history taking will have been inadequate and previous records may be unavailable. In these circumstances, potentially dangerous situations may surface for the first time during the recovery period.

Surgery for Trauma

1. *Full stomach.* Patients requiring emergency surgery following trauma must be assumed to have a full stomach. Efforts to empty the stomach before or during surgery by passing a nasogastric tube or administering metoclopramide are not invariably successful, so these patients should be nursed on their side with a slight head-down tilt. Extubation should be delayed until consciousness has returned and the patient objects to the presence of the tube. Vomiting may be copious and powerful suction with wide-bore tubing must be close at hand.

2. *Head injury.* A delayed return of consciousness may be due to alcohol, hypoglycaemia or head injury. If the history suggests the possibility of a head injury, regular neurological assessment using the Glasgow coma scale (see page 127) is recommended.

   Opiate administration should be avoided if possible as it will:

   (a) Depress the level of consciousness.

   (b) Depress respiration.

   (c) Interfere with examination of the pupils by causing constriction.

   Codeine phosphate is a suitable alternative without these disadvantages. If pain is inadequately controlled by codeine phosphate and more potent opiates are considered necessary, they should be administered intravenously in small increments until the minimal effective dose has been given.

3. *Associated injuries* may complicate the presenting surgical problem, for

example:

(a) Fractured ribs and the possibility of pneumothorax or haemothorax (page 78). Recovery staff must be alert to the possibility of tension pneumothorax (page 79) developing rapidly, especially if intermittent positive pressure ventilation is being used.

(b) Ruptured spleen causing persistent hypovolaemia.

(c) Fractured pelvis causing haematuria or anuria.

4. *Hypovolaemia.* Blood loss is frequently underestimated following trauma, particularly if there have been large scalp wounds or fractures of the long bones or pelvis. If signs of hypovolaemia develop post-operatively (i.e. pallor, collapsed veins, weak thready pulse, increasing heart rate, decreasing blood pressure and oliguria), intravenous fluid replacement must be accelerated using, if necessary, CVP measurements to guide therapy.

Surgery in the Accident Department

The patient must be assumed to have a full stomach and recover from anaesthesia in the lateral position with head-down tilt and suction to hand.

Following recovery from general anaesthesia, the patient must remain under observation in the accident department for at least 2h, during which time recovery staff must satisfy themselves that the patient is fully conscious, that his movements are co-ordinated and that he is to be escorted home by a responsible adult. Patients who have been intubated are only allowed home provided there has been no evidence of laryngeal stridor in the 2h following extubation. If suxamethonium (succinylcholine) has been used, the patient should be advised to restrict activity during the following 24h to minimise muscle pains. The dangers of taking alcohol, driving, cooking or operating machinery during the next 24h must be stressed, preferably in writing. An adequate supply of analgesics should be provided if post-operative pain is likely.

GASTROENTEROLOGY

Endoscopy

The incidence of perforation of the oesophagus is negligible with the use of the fibre-optic endoscope. However, patients may be at risk of gastro-oesophageal reflux and aspiration into the lungs if they have a hiatus hernia and an incompetent cardia; it is therefore particularly important that they are kept on their side while recovering from anaesthesia. When an oesophageal stricture is bypassed by the insertion of a tube, e.g. the Celestin tube, the regurgitation of the stomach contents becomes more likely and recovery staff should identify those patients at risk.

Perforation of the oesophagus is more likely when a rigid oesophagoscope has been used and after the dilatation of strictures (particularly those which are malignant), and it may first become evident in the recovery room.

The patient may complain of pain in the chest, neck or epigastrium. If they also develop pyrexia, tachycardia, hypotension and subcutaneous emphysema, it is probable that the oesophagus has been perforated. An intravenous infusion should be started and a chest X-ray taken while definitive management is arranged. The patient must not be allowed oral fluids.

Upper Gastrointestinal Tract Bleeding

Following operations to arrest bleeding, problems may occur in the recovery period because:

1. Blood replacement may have been inadequate.
2. Complications of massive transfusion may arise (pages 104–110).
3. Further bleeding may occur. This may be either revealed (haematemesis, fresh blood draining from the nasogastric tube) or concealed. If signs of hypovolaemia (page 78) persist despite blood replacement, the surgeon must be informed without delay.

If surgery has been performed because of bleeding from oesophageal varices (e.g. porto-caval anastomosis or oesophageal transection), problems associated with liver dysfunction (page 152) may occur.

Surgery for Intestinal Obstruction or Peritonitis

Patients with these conditions can develop severe fluid and electrolyte disturbances which may not have been corrected by the time they reach the recovery unit. Hypovolaemia, hypokalaemia and metabolic acidosis are not uncommonly found and lead to poor peripheral perfusion, cardiovascular collapse, dysrhythmias and difficulty in reversing muscle relaxants. These problems are more dangerous in children, in whom fluid depletion is easily underestimated. The state of the peripheral circulation and measurements of central venous pressure, urine output, urea and electrolytes, together with blood gas analysis, will provide useful guides for the correction of these abnormalities.

Bowel Surgery

Neostigmine is sometimes avoided following bowel surgery because of the damage it may cause to anastomoses by stimulating gut contraction. In such patients elective post-operative ventilation is continued until the effects of muscle relaxants have been eliminated.

Other problems occasionally encountered following bowel surgery include:

1. *Hypokalaemia* following prolonged diarrhoea or vigorous bowel wash-out. This may cause difficulty with reversal of muscle relaxants or dysrhythmias. Intravenous potassium supplements may be required.
2. *Hypothermia* following prolonged bowel exposure (see page 100).
3. *Adrenocortical insufficiency* may develop in patients receiving prolonged steroid therapy for inflammatory diseases of the bowel (see page 147).
4. *Septicaemia* (see page 82) may occur with toxic megacolon seen in ulcerative colitis or following gall bladder surgery.
5. *Prolongation of muscle relaxants* owing to the administration of antibiotics (see pages 72–75).

ORTHOPAEDIC SURGERY

Plaster Casts

When handling freshly applied plaster of Paris the palms of the hands should be used rather than the fingers, as they may cause indentations and subsequent discomfort. The principles of plaster cast care will also apply to compression bandages. The limb should be elevated to aid venous drainage and to reduce any consequent swelling. It should be supported on a firm pillow until the cast is fully hardened. One or more fingers or toes should be exposed so that any of the following signs of circulatory impairment can be readily observed:

1. Blanching of skin.
2. Cyanosis – refer to a normal limb for comparison.
3. Prolonged circulatory filling time – assess after a brief period of compression with the fingers.
4. Fall in temperature.
5. Sensory impairment.

The cast margin should be checked to ensure that it is not causing undue pressure on the underlying tissues. This is of particular importance with lower-limb casts which may cause a local pressure injury to the lateral popliteal nerve as it crosses the neck of the fibula. Pressure on this nerve will cause foot drop. It is important to note possible unprotected bony prominences which may be present. Bleeding should be noted and outlined on the plaster, together with the exact time of marking. If any untoward signs are present, the orthopaedic surgeon should be notified without delay.

Plaster jackets enclosing the thorax can restrict respirations. Adequate respiratory function must be confirmed before the patient is allowed to leave the recovery unit.

Traction

Traction cannot be adequately applied using the standard recovery trolley. If it is essential to apply traction in the immediate post-operative period, the patient's own bed can be brought from the ward for this purpose. When heavy weights are used, elevation of the foot of the bed will be necessary.

Reduction of Fractures

When fractures have been manipulated, careful observation of the limb distal to the fracture is required so that vascular (see above) or neurological impairment will be swiftly identified.

Limbs and joints must be adequately supported in a comfortable position, and signs of persistent blood loss on dressings or plasters, in drainage bottles or by increasing limb girth, must all be identified. If blood loss is significant, it may need to be replaced.

Hip Operations

Hip operations such as pin and plating are frequently performed on the frail and elderly, who may present with associated conditions, e.g. dehydration, anaemia, chest infection. Blood loss can be heavy and close observation of the cardiovascular system is required. Further fluid replacement or blood transfusion may also be required. Central venous pressure measurements are a useful guide to transfusion requirements in patients with cardiac failure. Spinal and epidural anaesthesia are often used to reduce blood loss, but additional precautions are needed post-operatively following these techniques (pages 56 and 57).

The groin should be inspected to identify any damage to the vulva or scrotum caused by the central peg during surgery, and any extraneous plaster should be removed.

Because these patients frequently have atrophic skin, the rough canvas should be removed early and carefully from beneath them to avoid skin damage. Early transfer of these patients to their own bed in the recovery room is preferable to nursing them on firm trolleys.

Deep-vein thrombosis is common and increases the risk of subsequent pulmonary embolism; early mobilisation and physiotherapy are employed to prevent venous stasis and reduce the risk of these complications.

Following hip replacement, steps must be taken to prevent dislocation. This may be done by using an abduction (Charnley) pillow. A patient who remains in the recovery unit for several hours should be turned on to the operated side to take pressure off the sacrum.

Fractured Vertebrae

Unstable vertebral fractures may cause damage to the spinal cord unless extreme caution is exercised when the patient is moved. Flexion, extension and twisting movements of the spine must be avoided and any lifting of the patient must be undertaken gently, slowly and in a co-ordinated way, with the vertebrae supported along their entire length, either by a firm canvas or by an adequate number of assistants.

Fractures of the cervical vertebrae are generally stabilised by traction applied to skull calipers. When these patients have to be lifted, the anaesthetist's full attention will be required to ensure that the head and neck move as one with the rest of the body. As the patients cannot be turned on to their side in an emergency, extra care will be needed in keeping the airway clear, and observations must not be relaxed until patients are fully conscious and able to protect their own airways.

OBSTETRICS AND GYNAECOLOGY

Caesarean Section

There is a risk of inhaling gastric contents post-operatively until an effective cough reflex has returned. When surgery has been completed, the patient remains intubated and is nursed on her side with a head-down tilt until consciousness has returned and she starts to object to the presence of the tube. Only when the patient has demonstrated that she can protect her own airway can extubation be safely performed. The attendant should be able to tell the mother the sex and condition of her baby when asked.

When spinal or epidural anaesthesia has been used, a degree of residual motor, sensory and autonomic block must be expected post-operatively (pages 56 and 57).

Post-operative Complications

These include the following:

1. *Post-partum haemorrhage.* The perineal pad is inspected regularly for signs of blood loss, and the fundal height and degree of contraction are checked. Fundal massage and the administration of oxytocics may be required. Oxytocin may be preferred in the presence of hypertension since ergometrine can itself cause a further rise in blood pressure. When oxytocin is used, a continuous infusion may be needed because of its short duration of action. Blood replacement will be required if there is continued loss. It might also be wise to take blood samples for coagulation studies (page 108).
2. *Pre-eclamptic toxaemia.* Intense observations must be maintained post-operatively in patients with pre-eclamptic toxaemia as the signs of deteriora-

tion (increasing blood pressure, proteinuria, oedema and oliguria) must be detected and treated if convulsions are to be avoided (page 99).

Management includes:

(a) Avoidance of undue stimulation. It is preferable to transfer patients to a quiet, darkened room.
(b) Sedation with a continuous infusion of diazepam or chlormethiazole in addition to analgesics.
(c) Reduction of blood pressure, e.g. by an infusion of hydralazine titrated against the patient's response.
(d) Fluid restriction.
(e) Diuretics.

3. *Amniotic fluid embolism.* This rare condition may follow Caesarean section or normal delivery and is characterised by a sudden onset of respiratory insufficiency and cardiovascular collapse. There is persistent bleeding with defective coagulation owing to disseminated intravascular coagulation (page 107).

Treatment consists of cardiovascular and respiratory support. Blood samples are taken for coagulation studies and the appropriate replacement therapy is given under the guidance of an experienced haematologist.

Evacuation of Retained Products of Conception; Suction Termination of Pregnancy

Perineal pads should be checked regularly for signs of continued bleeding. Further ergometrine or oxytocin should be given if required and hypovolaemia prevented by intravenous fluids or blood, if necessary.

A careful, understanding approach is needed for all patients after termination of pregnancy as emotional distress is common.

A perforated uterus must be suspected if there is:

1. Increasing pulse rate.
2. Decreasing blood pressure.
3. Pallor.
4. Inappropriate abdominal pain.

The surgeon must be informed without delay.

Laparoscopy

During this operation large volumes of carbon dioxide are insufflated into the peritoneal cavity. Although much of this is released at the end of the procedure, the abdomen may remain distended and pain and restlessness are common. Early administration of analgesics may be required.

Hysterectomy

Post-operative haemorrhage may complicate this operation so that close observation of the cardiovascular system and regular inspection of the wound dressing or pad must be undertaken. Vaginal packing may be required. If the ligature on the uterine pedicle slips, haemorrhage may be brisk and adequate blood replacement is required before further surgery.

When regional anaesthesia has been used, post-operative hypotension may occur but, provided peripheral perfusion is adequate and hypovolaemia is avoided, the blood pressure may be allowed to rise slowly as sympathetic tone returns (pages 56–57).

EAR, NOSE AND THROAT SURGERY

Tonsillectomy

Following surgery, patients are placed in the 'tonsillar position' to allow optimal drainage of blood and secretions. The patient is turned well over on to one side with a pillow under the lower shoulder and the head down (see Figure 5.1). An oral airway is inserted until the patient is conscious.

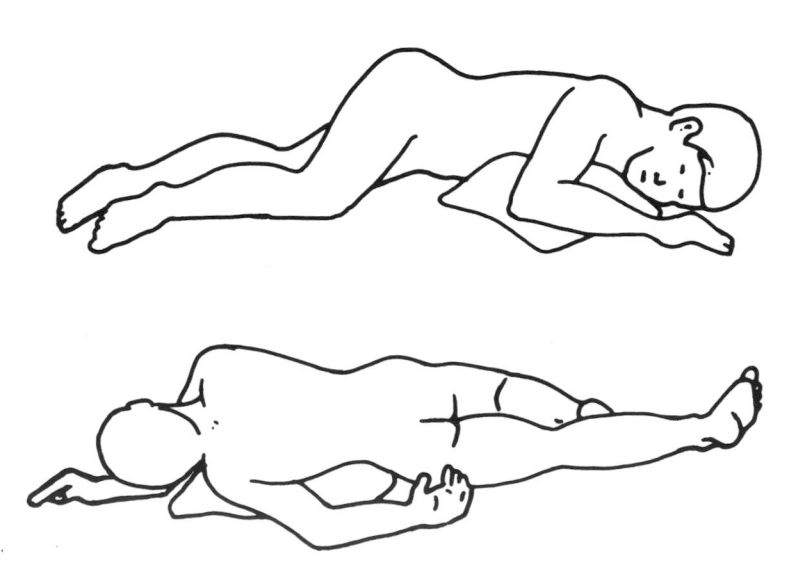

Figure 5.1 The 'tonsillar' position

Blind suction is avoided, if possible, as it may disturb clots of blood or displace ligatures, and cause further haemorrhage.

Post-operative haemorrhage is a serious complication which may rapidly lead to hypovolaemia if it is not detected early. It must be remembered that visible haemorrhage may represent only a small percentage of the blood lost, since much of the blood will be swallowed. Signs of persistent haemorrhage include:

1. Increased drainage of blood from the mouth.
2. Coughing and spitting of blood.
3. Frequent swallowing, sometimes followed by vomiting of blood.
4. Pallor.
5. Poor peripheral perfusion.
6. Increasing pulse rate.
7. Falling blood pressure.

If these signs occur, blood should be taken for cross-matching, an intravenous infusion established, and the surgeon and anaesthetist informed without delay, as further surgery may be required.

Laryngoscopy

The patient should be closely observed until the gag or cough reflexes return. The 'tonsillar position' is used until the patient is fully conscious. If a local anaesthetic has been applied topically during this procedure, the patient should not be allowed oral fluids for 4 h. Recovery may be accompanied by:

1. Violent coughing and dyspnoea.
2. Laryngospasm.
3. Stridor.
4. Bleeding, especially if a biopsy has been performed.

Humidified oxygen and resting the voice may help minimise problems. If stridor is marked, the patient should be given a helium–oxygen mixture (80% helium and 20% oxygen) to breathe. This will reduce the work of breathing, relieve the patient's anxiety and frequently allow the stridor to disappear.

Tracheostomy

The recovery-room staff should be forewarned of the arrival of any patient who has had a tracheostomy and should know the reason why the operation was necessary. The following should be readily available:

1. A range of tracheostomy tubes and a tracheal dilator.
2. Adequate suction.
3. Ambu bag.
4. Suitable catheter mounts.
5. Tracheostomy oxygen mask.

Immediate complications of tracheostomy may include:

1. *Obstruction of the tube* by blood or secretions. Suctioning should be carried out in a sterile manner using a disposable soft suction catheter with an air control port. Viscid secretions can be reduced by humidifying the inspired air or oxygen since the normal humidifying mechanisms of the upper airway have been bypassed (see page 31).

2. *Displacement of the tube.* The tracheostomy tube is secured in theatre using a double tie with reef knots. It should be sufficiently tight so that two fingers may just be inserted under the tape. If it is too loose, the tube may be expelled by coughing. This is a potential disaster as the tissue planes may move relative to one another. It can then be very difficult or impossible to replace the tracheostomy tube. After the tube has been in place for several days, a sinus forms. Removing and changing the tube is then relatively easy.

3. *Bleeding around wound edges,* which may require dressing changes.

Constant reassurance by recovery staff will be required as patients who have undergone tracheostomy may be very frightened and are unable to speak. Questions should be worded accordingly.

Operations on the Nose

Until fully conscious, these patients should remain in the "tonsillar" position to allow free drainage of blood and mucosal fluid (see Figure 5. 1). Once consciousness has been regained, the semi-Fowler's position (Figure 5.2) can be adopted to improve venous drainage and decrease local oedema.

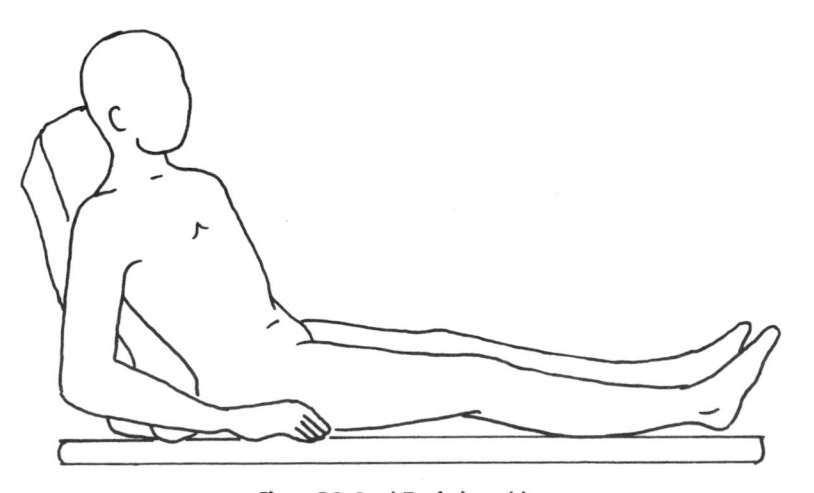

Figure 5.2 Semi-Fowler's position

A nasal pack is frequently inserted and held in place by taping it to the external nares. Its position should be checked and the amount of drainage noted. It is important that the pack should remain in this position as any movement into the post-nasal space may lead to subsequent airway obstruction.

Close observation must be maintained for signs of continued blood loss, much of which may trickle down the posterior pharyngeal wall and be swallowed (see Tonsillectomy, page 120).

These patients sometimes become confused and delirious post-operatively, possibly because of feelings of panic due to nasal obstruction. They may forget to mouth breathe and try to remove the packs by every means they can. They should be reminded to breathe through the mouth and gently reassured. A Guedel airway may be a useful means of keeping the mouth open during this phase (page 25).

When plaster of Paris has been applied to the nose following the reduction of fractured nasal bones, care must be taken to ensure that the patient does not roll over on to the nose and distort or displace the splint.

Hypotensive anaesthesia is frequently used for rhinoplasty. A degree of residual hypotension may persist into the post-operative period. Provided peripheral perfusion is adequate and hypovolaemia is avoided, blood pressure is allowed to rise slowly as the hypotensive agents are eliminated (page 145).

Middle-ear Surgery

Hypotensive techniques are frequently employed for middle-ear surgery and the post-operative nursing care is as outlined on page 145.

A pressure bandage is usually applied at the end of surgery. The patient lies on the unoperated side and the dressing is inspected frequently for signs of bleeding. This can be a problem if the blood pressure is allowed to rise too quickly after hypotensive anaesthesia.

Restlessness and vertigo frequently occur, particularly if there has been direct vestibular stimulation. These may be worse if the patient sits up. The patient is encouraged to remain quiet and still, and lie with a single pillow. Anti-emetics should be given.

As the facial nerve may be damaged during surgery, its integrity should be confirmed by checking that there is full movement of the facial muscles. This may be done by asking the patient to show their teeth or smile.

THYROID SURGERY

Airway Problems

Airway problems may be caused by:

1. *Obstruction* owing to formation of a haematoma which compresses the trachea (bleeding is usually from a branch of the superior thyroid artery). Pressure on the trachea can be relieved by removing the skin clips or sutures and evacuating the haematoma. It may be necessary to do this immediately without waiting for a surgeon. If this is unsuccessful, endotracheal intubation

is required; however, this may be difficult if the trachea is displaced, and a tracheostomy may have to be performed.

2. *Damage to recurrent laryngeal nerves.* This should be suspected if the vocal cords were not seen to move at extubation. It may be noted early in recovery by asking the patient to answer questions. If the recurrent laryngeal nerves are damaged, hoarseness or whispering will be evident. In more severe cases there may be stridor, and if both nerves are damaged bilateral abductor paralysis can cause obstruction of the airway, in which case re-intubation will be required. Damage to the cords is more likely following surgery for malignancy or in repeat operations.

3. *Collapsed trachea (tracheomalacia).* This may only become evident following extubation and may first be noticed in the recovery room. It is a rare complication and tends to occur when a very large thyroid has been removed. Reintubation will be required until more definitive management can be arranged.

Thyroid Crisis or Storm

Thyroid crisis or storm is rarely seen when the patient is adequately treated with antithyroid drugs pre-operatively and made euthyroid. The presenting features include tachycardia, hypertension, pyrexia, dyspnoea, confusion, dilated pupils and agitation. Management should be started without delay and should include:

1. Intravenous fluid replacement.
2. Oxygen therapy and possibly artificial ventilation.
3. Potassium iodide.
4. α- and β-blockade.
5. Cooling by tepid sponging and fanning.
6. Hydrocortisone.
7. Sodium bicarbonate to correct metabolic acidosis.
8. Sedation.

Once the condition has been stabilised, the patient's transfer to an intensive-care unit will be required for further management.

DENTAL AND FACIOMAXILLARY SURGERY

Post-operative Bleeding

Because continued bleeding within the mouth is common, it is particularly important that these patients are nursed on their side with a slight head-down tilt until they regain consciousness, so that blood does not pool in the pharynx.

A dental mouth pack may be in place at the end of surgery. This must not be allowed to obstruct the airway. Complete respiratory obstruction has been recorded when, unknown to the recovery staff, a pharyngeal pack was inadvertently left in place following extubation.

Persistent bleeding may require further surgical intervention. It is particularly dangerous if the blood is being swallowed as this may go unnoticed (see 'Tonsillectomy', page 120). Gentle suction with a soft suction catheter may be required. This can be conveniently applied via a nasopharyngeal airway or via a shortened nasotracheal tube pulled back so that its tip lies in the pharynx and with a safety pin through it at the nares.

Wiring of the Jaw

Following the reduction of mandibular fractures, facial bone reconstructions and mandibular osteotomies, stabilising wires (usually two or more on either side) are inserted to hold the jaw in a fixed position. Recovery staff should know the position of these wires as they may have to cut them if respiratory obstruction or vomiting occurs. Wire cutters should accompany the patient from the operating theatre and be readily available.

A tongue switch may also be inserted to allow the tongue to be pulled forwards should it obstruct the airway.

Vomiting is particularly hazardous when the jaws are wired, and the prophylactic use of anti-emetics can be useful. Suction can be applied via a nasopharyngeal airway.

Fracture of the Zygomatic Arch

Following reduction of the fracture, the patient is nursed with the affected side uppermost to avoid pressure on the fracture side.

Mentally Handicapped Patients

Mentally handicapped patients, both adults and children, who require dental treatment under general anaesthesia, need great care during the recovery period. The early administration of analgesics is helpful. As a significant number of these patients will be carriers of the Hepatitis B antigen, appropriate precautions should be taken to avoid contamination with their blood or saliva.

OPHTHALMIC SURGERY

Although some ophthalmic surgery is carried out under general anaesthesia, an increasing number of patients receive local anaesthesia. They embrace the extremes of age and include a high proportion of diabetics. As their sight is impaired, frequent explanations and quiet reassurance from the nursing staff will aid smooth recovery.

Position

Until they are fully conscious, patients should be nursed in the lateral position on the unaffected side. This will reduce the likelihood of direct pressure being applied to the eye, and should vomiting occur, the operated eye will not be contaminated.

Intra-ocular Pressure (IOP)

Vomiting, coughing and straining can all cause an unwanted rise in IOP. The pharynx is thoroughly suctioned prior to extubation to minimise pharyngeal stimulation during recovery. Anti-emetic and antitussive agents can be employed prophylactically to reduce the incidence of vomiting and coughing.

Pupil Size

This may be affected by eye drops given before or during surgery, including:

1. Mydriatics, e.g. cyclopentolate and phenylephrine, used to dilate pupils for retinal detachment surgery.
2. Miotics, e.g. pilocarpine, used to constrict pupils in glaucoma.

Analgesia

Pain is seldom severe after ophthalmic surgery except following correction of squint and retinal detachment. Children should be restrained from removing dressings and their co-operation sought by gentle persuasion.

Drug Interactions

Staff should be aware of drugs used in ophthalmology which may influence the patient's recovery. These include:

1. Ecothiopate, an anticholinesterase used in the treatment of glaucoma which will cause prolonged neuromuscular block if suxamethonium (succinylcholine) has been used.
2. Timolol, a β-blocking drug used in the treatment of glaucoma, can cause bradycardia.

NEUROSURGERY

Following neurosurgery, changes in intracranial pressure may occur which may be life-threatening if they go undetected. In specialised neurosurgical units, direct intracranial-pressure monitoring may be employed. Elsewhere, reliance must be placed in frequent clinical observations which may reflect intracranial events.

For this reason, patients who have undergone craniotomy or who have received a head injury, require more detailed post-operative monitoring than others. In addition to the standard observations of pulse, blood pressure and respiratory rate, regular examinations of the pupils and level of consciousness must be continued even after the effects of anaesthesia have apparently worn off. A neurological observation chart based on the Glasgow Coma Scale (see Figure 5.3, *overleaf*) provides a convenient way of recording these observations.

The following signs reflect intracranial events which may require intervention and should be brought to the attention of the neurosurgeon:

1. Deterioration in the level of consciousness.
2. Lateralising signs, especially pupillary dilation.
3. Rising blood pressure accompanied by falling pulse rate (Cushing's ischaemic reflex).
4. Changes in the respiratory pattern such as irregular breathing or a slowing of the respiratory rate.

It may become necessary to reduce intracranial pressure during the recovery period. The following methods are available:

1. Intravenous mannitol 0.25–0.5 g/kg over 30 min.
2. Intravenous dexamethasone 10 mg.
3. Intravenous frusemide (furosemide) 20–40 mg.
4. Intubation followed by controlled hyperventilation to maintain $PaCO_2$ at between 3.3 kPa and 4 kPa. A neurological assessment should be made before sedatives or muscle relaxants are given since these drugs mask the signs of rising intracranial pressure.

Recovery staff must be alert for any factors which may cause an undesirable rise in intracranial pressure in the post-operative period. These include:

1. Hypoxia and hypercarbia owing to respiratory obstruction or ventilatory impairment.
2. Increased venous pressure owing to coughing or straining, the head-down position or circulatory overload.
3. Hypertension or hypotension sufficient to interfere with autoregulation of cerebral blood supply.

Care in the post-operative period should therefore be directed towards:

1. *Ensuring adequate respiration:*
   (a) Careful attention to maintenance of a clear airway.
   (b) Administration of oxygen.
   (c) Blood-gas analysis. If hypoxia or hypercarbia occur, controlled ventilation may be required.

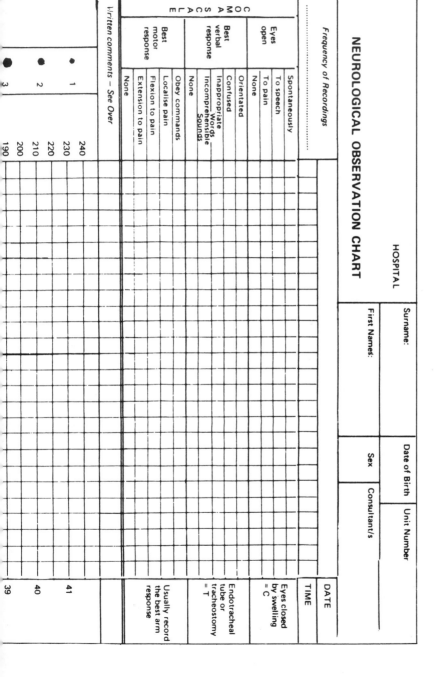

NEUROLOGICAL OBSERVATION CHART

HOSPITAL

Surname:		Date of Birth	Unit Number
First Names:		Sex	Consultant/s

Frequency of Recordings		DATE
		TIME

Eyes open	Spontaneously		Eyes closed by swelling = C
	To speech		
	To pain		
	None		

Best verbal response	Orientated		Endotracheal tube or tracheostomy = T
	Confused		
	Inappropriate Words		
	Incomprehensible Sounds		
	None		

Best motor response	Obey commands		Usually record the best arm response
	Localise pain		
	Flexion to pain		
	Extension to pain		
	None		

C O M A   S C A L E

Written comments – See Over

240
230
220
210
200
190

1 ·
2 ·
3 ●

39
40
41

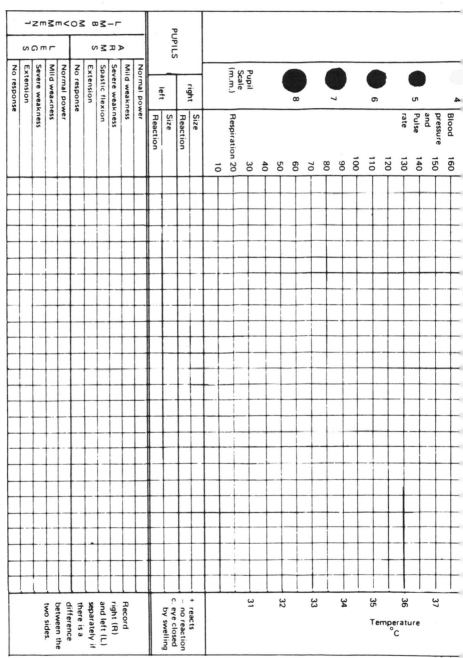

Figure 5.3 Neurological observation chart

2. *Avoidance of increased venous pressure:*
   (a) Patients should be nursed in a slight head-up position to encourage venous drainage.
   (b) Cautious intravenous fluid administration to avoid circulatory overload.
   (c) Prevention of coughing and straining. If an oropharyngeal airway or endotracheal tube causes irritation it should be taken out or the patient adequately sedated. Secretions must be promptly removed by suction catheter.
3. *Avoidance of excessive hypertension.* Hypotensive agents must be used with extreme caution following neurosurgery. Hypertension may be a sign of Cushing's ischaemic reflex and reducing the blood pressure may further prejudice brain-stem perfusion; consequently, investigation, e.g. brain scan or angiography, should precede treatment. Hypertension is frequently seen after aneurysm surgery with induced hypotension. Injudicious hypotensive therapy may cause vasospasm of the feeding vessels when the blood pressure falls, with resulting hemiparesis.

   In extreme cases, where hypotensive therapy is unavoidable, the patient should be transferred to an intensive-therapy unit since continuous blood-pressure monitoring is essential.

Temperature changes. Recovery from neurosurgery may be characterised by a disturbed body-temperature regulation. Constant monitoring and correction, if necessary, are required.

Hyperthermia may follow surgery in the region of the temperature-regulating centre in the hypothalamus, whereas hypothermia may result from prolonged anaesthesia and active cooling. Shivering should be avoided since this causes an increase in oxygen requirements. Sedation and controlled ventilation may be necessary to prevent this.

Convulsions may result from cerebral damage or oedema and should be managed in the standard way (see page 101).

THORACIC SURGERY

Bronchoscopy

The anaesthetic technique should provide a rapid return of the cough reflex post-operatively. If, however, topical or local anaesthesia has been used, the full return of reflexes may take several hours. The patient should be nursed in the lateral head-down position.

Post-operative complications include:

1. Laryngospasm (see page 68).
2. Laryngeal oedema, especially in children (see pages 69 and 138).
3. Bleeding. If this is severe, the surgeon and the anaesthetist must be informed. Treatment may include the introduction of an endobronchial blocker into the

affected lung and ventilation of the other lung via an endotracheal tube.

4. Perforation of the bronchus. The presenting features may include dyspnoea, retrosternal pain or surgical emphysema. The surgeon should be informed if perforation of the bronchus is suspected.

THORACOTOMY

Chest Drains

Following thoracic surgery, chest drains are usually inserted to enable air and fluid, including blood, to escape from the pleural cavity. They are normally positioned as follows:

1. Apical or upper drain to facilitate drainage of air.
2. Posterior or lower drain to facilitate drainage of blood.

A number of drainage systems are in use:

1. The simple underwater seal drainage bottle (Figure 5.4).
2. The Heimlich flutter valve – a disposable valve which allows air or blood to escape outwards but prevents air from re-entering the pleural cavity.
3. The Pleurevac system – a sterile disposable plastic unit.

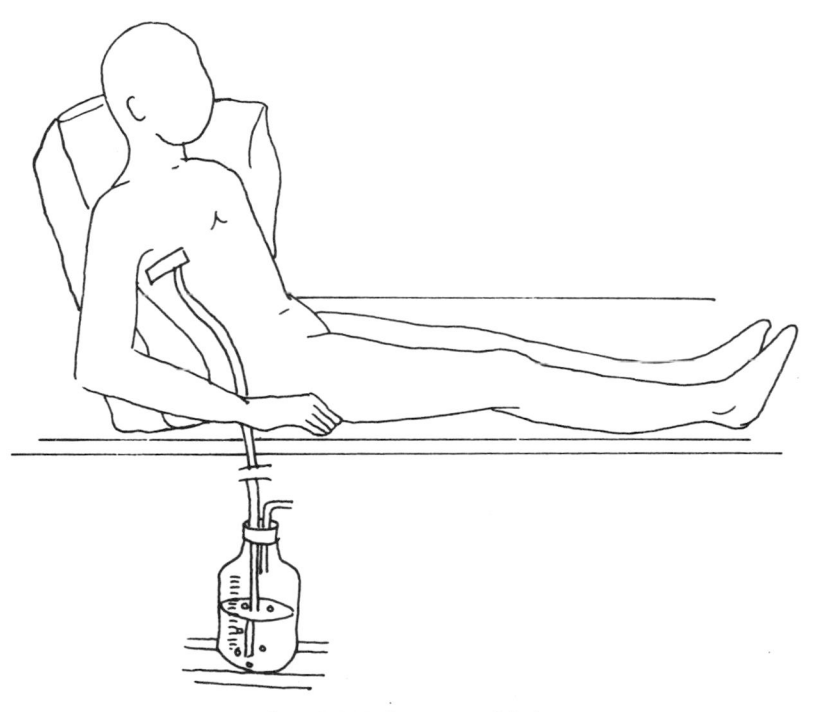

Figure 5.4 Underwater seal drain

Drainage through an underwater seal can be aided by attaching a mechanical pump (e.g. the Roberts pump) to the open end to provide continuous suction. The use of a suction pump is not advised following pneumonectomy as it may lead to gross mediastinal shift.

If the drainage tube is patent, the meniscus in the tube should rise and fall in time with respiration, and this should be checked regularly. If the tube becomes blocked, it may be cleared by 'milking' it with roller clamps, in the direction away from the patient.

Fluid from the drainage bottle must not be allowed to re-enter the pleural cavity; this can be ensured by keeping the bottle on the floor beneath the patient's bed. The tubing must be double clamped when the patient is being moved.

The volume of fluid escaping is measured using graduations on the side of the bottle. Changes in the fluid level should be recorded. There should be inter- mittent bubbling of air through the underwater seal, in time with respiration. Continuous bubbling throughout the respiratory cycle in a ventilated patient is indicative of a bronchopleural leak and the tidal volume may need to be in- creased.

The patient should be nursed in the supine position with gradual elevation to 45° as normal reflexes and consciousness return. This will aid lung expansion and facilitate fluid drainage.

X-ray

When the initial assessment of the patient has been completed, an X-ray of the chest should be taken in order to:

1. Confirm that re-expansion of the lungs has occurred.
2. Check the position of the mediastinum.
3. Exclude pneumothorax.
4. Ascertain the position of the chest drains and CVP catheter.
5. Reveal hidden bleeding.

Respiratory System

If the patient has been extubated, humidified oxygen should be given by face mask and adequate respiratory function confirmed using blood-gas analysis, if necessary. Deep breathing and coughing are encouraged to prevent lung infec- tions. The patient is best nursed in a sitting position to allow optimal movement of the diaphragm. Bronchial secretions can be copious and the trachea may need frequent aspiration. Adequate analgesia is essential and epidural narcotics or the intrapleural infusion of local anaesthetic may be the methods of choice (pages 57 and 61).

If the patient requires a period of elective post-operative ventilation, endo- tracheal suction should take place regularly. It is important that the catheter tip passes beyond the end of the endotracheal tube and enters each bronchus in turn.

Cardiovascular System

Blood loss may be extensive during thoracotomy and may continue post-operatively. Blood transfusion should be given as indicated by the clinical findings and not simply by the amount of blood lost in the chest drains.

Hypothermia

Heat loss during surgery may be considerable and hypothermia is managed as previously described (page 100).

Pain Relief

The importance of adequate pain relief after thoracic surgery cannot be over emphasised Such surgery is potentially extremely painful and if analgesia is inadequate the patient will not breathe sufficiently, cough or co-operate with the physiotherapist. The patient should be alert and pain-free when he leaves the recovery unit and, thereafter, analgesia should be matched to his individual requirements.

VASCULAR SURGERY

Note: The post-operative recovery of patients who have undergone the surgical repair of an aortic aneurysm is described here, although the same general principles apply to other forms of vascular surgery.

Patients requiring aortic surgery are usually elderly, with generalised arterial disease, so that a history of hypertension and myocardial ischaemia is common. Post-operatively they are frequently transferred directly to an intensive-care unit where elective ventilation may be continued until cardiovascular stability returns. If, however, intensive care facilities are not available, patients must be monitored closely in the recovery room until they are ready to return to the ward.

Oxygen therapy is given routinely and respiratory performance monitored by blood-gas analysis. Arterial blood samples should not, however, be taken from the femoral artery as grafts may be damaged.

The following problems may be encountered:

1. *Hypertension.* This is frequently seen post-operatively, possibly owing to renin release after aortic cross-clamping. It will put an unnecessary strain on the graft and is particularly dangerous in patients with myocardial ischaemia. Active measures are taken to reduce the blood pressure to normal values (see page 83).
2. *Hypotension.* This is commonly due to inadequate blood replacement. Bleeding may continue post-operatively; the drainage bottles must be care-

fully watched, and blood loss measured and replaced. It must be remembered that concealed bleeding may be significant. The pulse-rate and central-venous-pressure measurements provide a useful guide to replacement.

3. *Oliguria.* Renal perfusion may have been impaired by cross-clamping of the aorta or by hypovolaemia. Urine output is monitored and maintained above a minimum of 0.5 ml/(kg h) (see page 110). A 'renal' dose of dopamine (2–3 µg/(kg min)) is often given prophylactically.

4. *Hypothermia.* This may be due to prolonged bowel exposure and large transfusions of cold blood, and will result in vasoconstriction with further hypertension, myocardial depression and irritability (see page 100).

5. *Failure of coagulation.* Following intra-operative heparinisation and the transfusion of large volumes of blood, coagulation may be impaired post-operatively. If persistent bleeding is a problem, blood samples are taken for coagulation studies and the appropriate replacement therapy given (see page 108).

6. *Electrolyte imbalance.* This may be due to massive blood transfusion, diuretic therapy or hypothermia. Blood is taken in the early post-operative period for electrolyte estimation so that abnormalities can be detected and corrections made where necessary.

7. *Metabolic acidosis due to impaired circulation in the lower limbs when the aorta is cross-clamped.* This may result in impaired myocardial contraction and difficulty in reversing non-depolarising muscle relaxants. Sodium bicarbonate is used to correct severe degrees of metabolic acidosis using the formula

$$\tfrac{1}{3} \times \text{Body weight (kg)} \times \text{Base deficit} = \text{Amount of sodium bicarbonate required (mmol)}$$

This is usually given in small increments, and progress is monitored by serial measurements to prevent overcorrection.

8. *Thrombus formation.* The limbs must be frequently inspected for signs of impaired circulation (pallor, cyanosis, drop in temperature), and the pulses felt (see page 17). A Doppler ultrasonic device may prove useful in detecting thrombus formation. The surgeon must be informed if the peripheral circulation appears impaired as further surgery may be indicated.

Pain Relief

Continuous analgesia via an epidural catheter is frequently used following aortic surgery. The catheter must be positioned pre-operatively before the patient is heparinised to avoid the possibility of neurological damage due to haematoma formation. This method of pain relief has the additional advantage of improving blood flow due to sympathetic blockade, but recovery staff must be aware of the further implications (see pages 56 and 57).

Intramuscular opiates will be poorly absorbed if tissue perfusion is impaired post-operatively; small increments given intravenously will be more effective.

GENITO-URINARY SURGERY

Prostatectomy

Most prostatic surgery is performed via the transurethral route using a resecto-scope. As many patients who require this type of surgery are old and may have significant respiratory or cardiac disease, epidural or spinal anaesthesia is frequently employed.

Bladder Irrigation

In order to prevent clots of blood blocking the urinary catheter following prosta-tectomy, the bladder is continuously irrigated. Warming the irrigation fluid will minimise heat loss and vasoconstriction The volume of irrigation fluid instilled into the bladder and the volume drained must be recorded, and any discrepancy noted. Such discrepancies may occur if the bladder has been perforated.

Bladder distension may cause patients to feel that they need to micturate. They may worry that they will become incontinent, and constant reassurance is required.

The abdomen should be inspected periodically for signs of excessive bladder distension. Manual compression of the bladder may aid drainage, especially following spinal or epidural anaesthesia. If the catheter becomes blocked by clots, these should be removed without delay using a bladder syringe. If this is difficult or incomplete, the patient must return to the theatre for operative removal of the clots.

Fluid Balance

Large volumes of fluid may be absorbed from the prostatic bed during and after surgery, with the danger of circulatory overload. As the absorbed fluid may contain little sodium, a dilutional hyponatraemia can result. This is characterised by restlessness and confusion, leading to convulsions and coma. Treatment is with hypertonic saline (sodium chloride 1.8%) and diuretics.

Blood Pressure

Hypotensive anaesthesia is frequently employed to reduce bleeding during pros-tatectomy. The blood pressure should be allowed to rise slowly during the post-operative period as a sudden rise in pressure may provoke brisk haemorrhage and increase the chances of clot formation. As blood loss may continue during the recovery period, the circulating volume must be maintained with intra-venous fluids (page 145). Sodium chloride 0.9% is suitable, as it helps to maintain sodium levels. If bleeding is excessive, blood transfusion will be required. Traction on the catheter will exert pressure on the prostatic bed and aid the control of bleeding. The surgeon should be kept informed of persistent bleeding as further surgery may be indicated.

Perforated Bladder

This may follow prostate or bladder surgery and must be suspected if the following occur:

1. Increasing pulse rate.
2. Hypotension.
3. Abdominal pain and tenderness. This may be masked following spinal or epidural anaesthesia. There may be upper abdominal or shoulder pain owing to irritation of the diaphragm with irrigation fluids.
4. Abdominal distension with absent bowel sounds.
5. Continuous small deficits in bladder irrigation fluid measurements. The irrigation should be stopped and the surgeon informed without delay.

Disseminated Intravascular Coagulation (DIC)

DIC or fibrinolysis may follow prostatectomy owing to the absorption of prostatic tissue into the circulation. DIC will cause persistent bleeding and is diagnosed on the basis of the results of a clotting screen (page 108). The prostatic bed is sometimes perfused with a solution containing aminocaproic acid to prevent this complication.

Septic Shock

The absorption of endotoxins or bacteria into the circulation at prostatectomy may lead to septic shock, which is characterised by pyrexia, tachycardia, hypotension and a weak thready pulse. Vigorous antibiotic therapy and intravenous fluid therapy will be required. If there is no improvement despite adequate hydration and the CVP is high, inotropic support with a dopamine infusion may be helpful. Urine output should be maintained above 0.5 ml/(kg h) using diuretics if necessary. Following initial resuscitation, transfer to an intensive-care unit is recommended.

Nephrectomy

Atelectasis of the lower lung may occur when this operation is performed with the patient on one side in the jack-knife position. Early post-operative physiotherapy with adequate analgesia will help re-expand the lung.

A post-operative chest X-ray is taken to exclude pneumothorax resulting from accidental damage to the pleura. Should a pneumothorax be found, it will be necessary to insert a chest drain with an underwater seal.

Circumcision

It is both easy and satisfying to provide excellent post-operative analgesia for children who undergo circumcision. Penile blocks and caudal epidural analgesia are equally safe and effective (pages 62 and 60).

PAEDIATRIC SURGERY

Post-operatively in paediatric patients, special attention must be paid, not only to maintaining adequate respiratory and cardiovascular function, but also to temperature regulation and fluid balance.

Maintenance of Airway and Adequacy of Ventilation

When assessing respiratory function in infants, as opposed to adults, it should be remembered that:

1. The ribs are horizontal and breathing is mainly diaphragmatic.
2. Respiratory rates of between 30 and 40 per minute are normal.
3. The narrowest point of the upper airway is at the cricoid cartilage.

Face masks and nasal cannulae are unsatisfactory in conscious patients, and if oxygen therapy is required, an incubator, tent or face tent should be used. An incubator is preferable for smaller infants as temperature, oxygen therapy and humidity are more easily controlled, but a tent is needed for larger infants.

The following may be required for airway management, and should be readily available:

1. A range of paediatric oral airways.
2. A range of anaesthetic face masks.
3. A range of endotracheal tubes and introducers (Table 5.1, *overleaf*). It may be wise for the paediatric anaesthetic circuit, laryngoscope, endotracheal tube and mask to accompany the patient from the operating theatre to the recovery unit.
4. Paediatric laryngoscope.
5. Paediatric anaesthetic circuit or Ambu bag so that assisted ventilation can be given either by face mask or via an endotracheal tube.
6. Fine suction catheters that can pass through endotracheal tubes.

The causes of respiratory inadequacy found in paediatric patients are essentially the same as those found in adults (see pages 70–79). Similarly, management is directed towards:

1. *Ensuring a clear airway* by inserting an oropharyngeal airway, supporting the jaw and removing any foreign matter by suction.
2. *Assisting inadequate respiratory efforts* by giving intermittent positive-pressure ventilation via a face mask and reservoir bag. This should take

precedence over attempts at intubation, which is seldom necessary and should only be attempted by those with adequate experience.

Table 5.1. Endotracheal tube sizes

Age (years)	Internal diameter of tube (mm)
Neonate	3.0
1	4.0
2	5.0
4	5.5
6	6.0
8	6.5
10	7.0
12	7.5

Tube length $oral = 12 + \dfrac{age}{2}$ (cm)

Tube length $nasal = 13.5 + \dfrac{age}{2}$ (cm)

Post-extubation Sub-glottic or Laryngeal Oedema

The incidence of this serious complication has been reduced by the use of endotracheal tubes made of non-irritant material, e.g. PVC, and of a size that allows a slight air leak. Oedema is more likely if there have been difficulties with intubation or if there is an upper respiratory tract infection; it must be recognised and treated promptly because of the danger of respiratory obstruction.

The *first signs* frequently appear within 2 h of extubation and include:

1. Inspiratory stridor.
2. Croupy cough.
3. Rib retraction.
4. Restlessness.
5. Pallor or cyanosis.

Treatment

This includes:

1. Oxygen.
2. Humidity.
3. Head-up position to increase venous drainage.
4. Diuretics.
5. Dexamethasone.
6. Antibiotics.
7. Nebulised adrenaline (racemic epinephrine).

The use of sedatives is not recommended. If this treatment is unsuccessful, intubation is required to bypass the obstruction.

Loose teeth present a frequent hazard and are best removed in a controlled way while the child is still unconscious in case they fall out during recovery and are inhaled. Teeth should be saved and returned to the ward with the patient for the attention of 'the tooth fairy'.

Maintenance of Adequate Cardiovascular Function

Although the same general principles of assessing cardiovascular function in adults (page 16) apply in paediatric patients, certain differences should be borne in mind:

1. The normal heart rate is faster (Table 5.2 and Figure 5.5, *overleaf*). This can conveniently be monitored using a precordial stethoscope which will, in addition, allow breath sounds to be heard.

Table 5.2. Relationship of heart rate to age

Age	Approximate heart rate (beats per minute)
Birth	140
1 month	130
1 year	120
2 years	110
4 years	100
8 years	90
12 years	80

2. The blood pressure is lower (Table 5.3). When measuring the blood pressure it is essential that the correct size of cuff is used (see Table 2.3). The blood pressure can be measured using a stethoscope on the brachial artery or with a suitable automatic device e.g. Dinamap.

3. The margin of safety following haemorrhage is less. Because of the small total blood volume, a comparatively small blood loss in absolute terms can represent a considerable proportion of the total circulating blood volume. Measuring blood loss must be precise and early fluid replacement will be required to prevent hypovolaemia.

Table 5.3. Relationship of blood pressure to age

Age	Approximate blood pressure (mmHg)
Birth	75/45
1 month	80/50
1 year	85/60
2 years	90/60
4 years	95/60
8 years	100/60
12 years	110/65

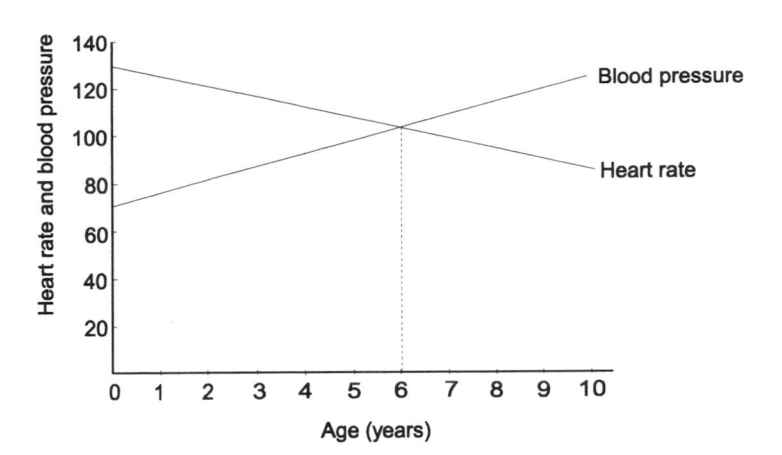

Figure 5.5 Relationship of heart rate and blood pressure with age. The systolic blood pressure gradually rises from 70 to 130. The heart rate falls from 130 to 70. At the age of 6 years the value of both is 100 appoximately

4. The heart is especially sensitive to vagally mediated bradycardia following upper-airway stimulation and suxamethonium (succinylcholine). The heart rate usually recovers quickly, but atropine may be required and should be readily available. Continuous ECG monitoring will give an early warning of changes of heart rate or rhythm, but it must be remembered that it indicates electrical activity and gives no indication of the mechanical efficiency of the heart.

Temperature Regulation

Small children have a greater tendency than adults to lose heat during surgery because:

1. They have a proportionally greater surface area to mass.
2. Their temperature-regulating centre is underdeveloped.
3. They have less subcutaneous fatty tissue.
4. Their ability to shiver, and so regenerate heat, is less well developed.

They are frequently cold when they arrive in the recovery room so it is particularly important that their temperature is monitored post-operatively. Low temperatures must be corrected before the patient is allowed to return to the ward (page 100).

Conversely, high temperatures may be found in children and these must also be detected and treated, as cerebral hypoxia or convulsions may follow (see page 101). A raised temperature may also indicate that the child is developing malignant hyperthermia (page 102).

Fluid Balance

In addition to the replacement of blood and fluids lost before and during surgery, the basic fluid maintenance requirements should be given to all children, except those undergoing very minor surgery, who may be expected to drink again soon after they recover from their anaesthetic.

Normal maintenance values (Table 5.4) can be used as a guideline, but must be adjusted according to individual circumstances, e.g. dehydration and pyrexia. Hartmann's solution or 0.9% sodium chloride should not normally be given; instead, dextrose/saline solutions (0.18% or 0.45% NaCl in 5% dextrose) should be used. If there has been a long period of starvation in the peri-operative period, hypoglycaemia may occur. This can be confirmed by using Dextrostix and treated with intravenous glucose.

Table 5.4. Maintenance intravenous fluid requirements

First month of life	6 ml/(kg h) (during the first week the requirements are less – multiply the age in days and divide by 7)
After the first month	
< 10 kg	4 ml/(kg h)
10–20 kg	3 ml/(kg h)
20–30 kg	2 ml/(kg h)
> 30 kg	1.5 ml/(kg h)

A reliable infusion site is essential and the cannula should be secured by adequate strapping and splinting in such a way that inspection of the puncture site and the rapid detection of the extravasation of infused solutions are possible. A butterfly needle is easily displaced and is not recommended for a prolonged infusion.

Some method of volume limitation should be used to prevent accidental overloading of the circulation, especially in infants and small children. The Metriset allows a convenient method of administration of small volumes of fluid and provides a degree of safety, as the chamber will require refilling periodically, but for greater reliability an infusion pump such as the IVAC is recommended.

References and Bibliography

Atkinson RS (1979). Post-operative care. In: Hewer CL, Atkinson RS (Eds), Recent Advances in Anaesthesia and Analgesia, No. 13. Churchill Livingstone, Edinburgh, pp. 185–197.

Atkinson RS, Rushman GB, Lee JA (1982). A Synopsis of Anaesthesia, 9th edn. Wright, Bristol.

Brown TCK, Fisk GC (1979). Anaesthesia for Children, Including Aspects of Intensive Care. Blackwell Scientific, Oxford, pp. 135–140.

Churchill-Davidson HC (Ed) (1978). A Practice of Anaesthesia, 4th edn. Lloyd-Luke, London.

Enderby GEH (1985). Hypotensive Anaesthesia. Churchill Livingstone, London.

Gothard JWW, Branthwaite MA (1982). Anaesthesia for Thoracic Surgery. Blackwell Scientific, London.

Hatch DJ (1981). Anaesthetic equipment for neonates and infants. Br J Hosp Med, 26, 84–88.

Jewkes D (1987). Anaesthesia for Neurosurgery. Clinical Anaesthesiology, Baillière Tindall, New York.

Miller RD (1981). Anaesthesia. Churchill Livingstone, New York.

Morrison JD, Mirakur RK, Craig HJL (1985). Anaesthesia for Eye, Ear, Nose and Throat Surgery. Churchill Livingstone, London.

Jackson RG, Gray TC (1981). Paediatric Anaesthesia: Trends in Current Practice. Butterworths, London.

Selwyn Crawford J (1984). Obstetric Analgesia and Anaesthesia. Churchill Livingstone, London.

Smith GB (1983). Ophthalmic Anaesthesia. Arnold, London.

Steward DJ (1979). Manual of Paediatric Anaesthesia. Churchill Livingstone, New York, Edinburgh, London.

Walters FJM, Nott MR (1977). The hazards of anaesthesia in the injured patient. Br J Anaesth, 49, 707–720.

Willatts SM, Walters FJM (1986). Anaesthesia and Intensive Care for the Neurosurgical Patient. Blackwell Scientific, London.

Chapter 6
PRE-EXISTING FACTORS AFFECTING RECOVERY

PREMEDICATION

The type and dosage of drugs given as premedication can influence recovery from anaesthesia in many ways:

1. *A relative overdose of depressant drugs relative to the patient's age and weight.* This is one of many causes of a delayed return of consciousness (page 93). This is particularly true when large doses of narcotic analgesic agents are given to the frail and elderly, but relative overdose may also follow benzodiazepine, phenothiazine or hyoscine (scopolamine) administration. Reversal of the effects of opiates can be achieved by intravenous naloxone (0.1–0.4 mg) or doxapram (50–100 mg).

2. *Benzodiazepines.* These can be reversed by the recently introduced specific antagonist flumazenil. Like naloxone, it should be administered slowly until the desired effect is obtained. The usual dose is 300–600 µg.

3. *Long-acting premedicating agents.* The action of some of these may persist into the post-operative period, especially if the surgical procedure is brief. Examples include droperidol and lorazepam.

4. *Anti-sialogogues.* When anti-sialogogues have been omitted, recovery may be accompanied by excessive salivation, especially following intubation, oral surgery and certain premedications, e.g. lorazepam. Frequent suction may be necessary to maintain a clear airway and to prevent coughing and laryngeal irritation.

ANAESTHETIC TECHNIQUE

Intravenous Induction Agents

When propofol has been used for induction of anaesthesia, recovery is generally rapid as the agent is quickly metabolised. This is obviously an advantage especially in patients who are having day surgery. However, if analgesics have not been given intra-operatively, they may be needed as soon as the patient awakes.

Long-acting Inhalational Agents

The higher the blood:gas solubility ratio of inhalational agents, the slower is their rate of elimination. Return of consciousness will therefore be prolonged following the use of the more soluble agents such as trichlorethylene and di-ethylether. Less soluble agents such as halothane, enflurane and isoflurane allow a more rapid recovery.

Analgesic and Relaxant Technique

A much lighter plane of anaesthesia can be achieved with a nitrous oxide–relaxant–hyperventilation technique with opiate supplements than by allowing a patient to breathe volatile agents spontaneously. Recovery of consciousness is correspondingly quicker.

Regional Anaesthesia

Patients who have been rendered pain-free by regional techniques, e.g. caudal anaesthesia, will tend to sleep peacefully once consciousness has returned, free of the restlessness and hypertension which characterise the patient in pain. This is especially valuable in children following painful operations such as circumcision. When spinal or epidural anaesthesia have been used, in addition to the sensory block, a degree of motor and autonomic block may persist into the post-operative period. It is important for recovery staff to be aware of this because:

1. The patient may be alarmed at his inability to move and will require reassurance.
2. Sudden changes in posture may cause hypotension.
3. Hypovolaemia must not be allowed to occur as compensatory vasoconstriction is impaired.
4. Urinary retention is common.

Brachial plexus block may persist well after completion of surgery and the arm may need to be supported in a sling for protection until motor function has returned. If the supraclavicular approach has been used, pneumothorax is a potential side-effect that may not become obvious until the patient is in the recovery room. Such patients may also notice voice changes owing to recurrent laryngeal nerve blockade.

Induced Hypotension

Deliberate hypotension used to facilitate surgery and reduce blood loss can be achieved in many ways including:

1. *Depression of myocardial contractility* (negative inotropic effect), e.g. by halothane, β-blocking agents.
2. *Sympathetic blockade* by ganglion-blocking agents, e.g. trimetaphan, or by spinal or epidural anaesthesia.
3. *Vasodilating drugs*, e.g. isoflurane, α-blocking agents, nitroprusside, nitro-glycerine.

Following the use of these techniques, patients may arrive in the recovery unit with some degree of residual hypotension. Providing there is no hypovolaemia and peripheral perfusion is good, the blood pressure can normally be allowed to rise slowly as the agents are eliminated. A sudden rise in blood pressure may provoke unwanted haemorrhage. These patients do not tolerate sudden changes in posture and, in particular, they should not sit up until the effects of the hypotensive agents have worn off. It should be remembered that patients who have received ganglion-blocking agents may have widely dilated pupils unresponsive to light.

If persistent or excessive hypotension occurs:

1. Give oxygen by face mask.
2. Elevate the foot of the bed to improve the venous return.
3. Increase the rate of intravenous fluid administration.

Subsequent treatment will depend on the mechanism of action of the drugs used and may consist of:

1. Positive inotropic agents, e.g. 10% calcium gluconate, up to 10 ml slowly i.v.
2. Direct-acting vasoconstrictors, e.g. methoxamine 20 mg diluted in 500 ml sodium chloride 0.9%.
3. Drugs combining both actions, e.g. ephedrine in increments of 5–10 mg i.v.

Ketamine

Patients who have been given ketamine may remain unconscious for several hours. To reduce emergence delirium, which is exacerbated by unwarranted stimulation, they should be nursed in a quiet corner of the recovery room until consciousness has returned. Disturbing hallucinations can be minimised by intravenous diazepam.

PRE-OPERATIVE DRUG THERAPY

Anti-hypertensive Agents

Drugs used to lower blood pressure may act either by reducing the tone in the peripheral vessels, e.g. guanethidine, methyldopa and ACE inhibitors, or by reducing the force of cardiac contraction, e.g. β-blockers:

1. *Drugs reducing peripheral vascular tone.* The ability of vessels to constrict in response to hypovolaemia or hypotension is impaired. Blood volume must be maintained post-operatively. Severe hypotension in the absence of hypovolaemia can be treated with direct-acting vasoconstricting agents such as methoxamine.
2. *β-blocking agents.* If severe bradycardia or hypotension occurs in patients on β-blockers, additional β-stimulation can be provided by an isoprenaline (isoproterenol) infusion under ECG monitoring. Circulating volume must be maintained.

Monoamine Oxidase Inhibitors (MAOIs)

Examples of MAOIs include pargyline, phenelzine and tranylcypromine.

Extreme care should be taken if using pethidine (meperidine) and morphine derivatives for post-operative analgesia in patients receiving MAOI therapy. Many reactions to such combinations have been reported, including:

1. Muscle twitching.
2. Hypotension.
3. Ataxia.
4. Cerebral excitation.
5. Coma.
6. Respiratory depression.

If no alternative method of post-operative analgesia is effective, a small test dose of pethidine, e.g. 5 mg, may be tried. If there is no abnormal reaction, further increments may be given at 5 min intervals until sufficient analgesia is produced.

Patients taking MAOIs may also develop marked hypertension if given pressor agents and care is thus recommended with:

1. Ephedrine.
2. Amphetamines.
3. L-dopa.

Adrenaline (epinephrine), however, is not harmful as it is metabolised by catechol-O-methyltransferase to monoamine oxidase.

Corticosteroids

The amount of hydrocortisone secreted in response to surgery may be 400 mg/day. Patients on long-term steroid therapy and those who have received a course of steroids within the previous 6 months can develop adrenocortical insufficiency in the immediate post-operative period. Such patients may be unable to respond to the stress of anaesthesia and surgery, and will require supplemental steroids.

Steroid cover in the form of hydrocortisone hemisuccinate 100 mg i.m. can be given with the premedication and repeated 6-hourly for 2 days following major surgery, and for 24 hours following minor surgery. For a very brief procedure a single injection should be sufficient.

The blood pressure should be carefully monitored following surgery in this group of patients since adrenocortical insufficiency may present as hypotension unexplained by other causes. Treatment is by a bolus of hydrocortisone 100–200 mg and intravenous fluids.

Insulin and Hypoglycaemic Agents

See under diabetes mellitus, page 154.

Anticoagulants

1. *Heparin.* This is used as a prophylaxis against deep-vein thrombosis and pulmonary embolism (see page 82). A dose of 5000 units subcutaneously before surgery should not cause bleeding problems post-operatively. Full anticoagulation with heparin, as used in cardiovascular surgery, will require reversal with protamine sulphate (page 107).
2. *Oral anticoagulants* (e.g. warfarin, phenindione). These are used prophylactically in patients with a history of:
   (a) Pulmonary embolism.
   (b) Recurrent thrombophlebitis.
   (c) Valve disease.
   (d) Valve replacement.

These patients are normally converted to treatment with intravenous heparin before surgery. Oral anticoagulant administration is then ceased. In an emergency, anticoagulation produced by warfarin may be reversed with a transfusion of fresh frozen plasma.

Diuretics

Patients with cardiac failure, ischaemic heart disease and hypertension may be receiving diuretic therapy. If potassium supplementation has been inadequate, hypokalaemia may result in:

1. Cardiac irregularities (page 86).
2. Prolonged neuromuscular block (pages 72–75).

In these patients, further intravenous potassium replacement will be required.

Antibiotics

Aminoglycoside antibiotics, such as gentamicin and neomycin, may occasionally prolong the neuromuscular blockade produced by non-depolarising relaxants. Full reversal should always be ensured before patients are allowed to leave the recovery room if they have received these agents. Intravenous calcium may be of value in speeding recovery from neuromuscular block in such patients.

Digoxin

The side-effects of digoxin treatment are greater if the patient is also hypo-kalaemic. If this occurs in the recovery period, signs of digoxin toxicity (especially dysrhythmias) may occur, and urgent intravenous potassium replacement is required.

If inotropic support becomes necessary in a patient already receiving digoxin, further digoxin is inadvisable as toxicity may occur. Dopamine or dobutamine are suitable alternatives.

RESPIRATORY DISEASE

Chronic Bronchitis

Patients with chronic bronchitis become insensitive to raised $PaCO_2$ levels and rely on a hypoxic drive to stimulate respiration. Uncontrolled oxygen therapy in the recovery period may decrease the normal respiratory drive and lead to hypoventilation. Graded concentrations of oxygen should be administered via a Venturi mask (Figure 2.12, page 32) starting with 24%, and progress monitored with a pulse oximeter or by serial blood gas estimations. If respiration is inadequate, doxapram, given either as a bolus or as a continuous infusion, may stimulate respiration, but intubation and controlled ventilation may be required until the effects of surgery and anaesthesia have worn off. If opiates are used for post-operative analgesia, extreme caution is needed as respiratory failure may be precipitated. Small intravenous increments should be titrated against the patient's response so as to avoid excessive administration. Alternatively, regional anaesthesia may enable adequate pain relief to be achieved without the need for opiates (pages 57 and 61).

In severe bronchitis, a period of elective ventilation in an intensive-care unit may be indicated, especially if there is a high abdominal or thoracic incision.

Asthma

Patients suffering from asthma must be particularly closely observed as episodes of bronchospasm may be precipitated by upper airway irritation or drugs (see page 76). If bronchospasm does occur, high concentrations of oxygen can, and should, be administered.

CARDIOVASCULAR DISEASE

Certain pre-operative factors are now recognised as being associated with an increased risk of ischaemia, infarction or death when patients undergo anaesthesia and surgery. In order of importance, these are:

1. A third heart sound or jugular venous distension, i.e. evidence of inadequately treated cardiac failure.
2. A myocardial infarction within the preceding six months.
3. Rhythms other than sinus or premature atrial contractions.
4. More than five ventricular ectopics per minute.
5. Age over 70 years.
6. Emergency surgery.
7. Aortic stenosis.
8. Poor general medical condition.

Coronary Artery Disease

When myocardial oxygen demand exceeds supply, myocardial ischaemia or infarction will result. Patients with coronary artery disease are particularly prone to develop this complication in the recovery room if:

1. Myocardial oxygen supply is reduced by hypoxaemia or by a diastolic pressure inadequate to perfuse the coronary arteries, or
2. Myocardial oxygen requirements are increased by excessive cardiac work load, e.g. hypertension, tachycardia, shivering.

Myocardial ischaemia is best prevented by:

1. Administration of oxygen.
2. Maintenance of pulse rate and blood pressure at normal pre-operative values.
3. Early and adequate pain relief.

Evidence of myocardial ischaemia can be demonstrated by the appearance of depressed ST segments on the ECG.

Hypertension

It is important for the recovery staff to know the pre-operative blood pressure and to relate post-operative measurements to this. Details of anti-hypertensive drug therapy must also be known (see page 146).

Patients with hypertension have a non-compliant circulation owing to athero-sclerotic changes in the vessel walls and anti-hypertensive therapy. Changes in circulating volume can result in extreme variations in blood pressure.

The principles of post-operative management include:

1. Frequent blood-pressure measurements and prompt correction of any major fluctuations.
2. Maintenance of normal circulating volume.
3. Adequate analgesia to prevent a hypertensive response to pain.

Cardiac Failure

The management of the patient with cardiac failure in the recovery period includes the following:

1. *Administration of oxygen.*
2. *Posture.* A trolley or bed which allows the patient to sit up should be available.
3. *Fluid restriction.* Intravenous fluids must be administered cautiously as circulatory overload can easily be precipitated. Central venous or pulmonary capillary wedge pressure measurements will provide a guide to fluid therapy.
4. *Inotropic support.* When inotropic support is required, digoxin or one of the more rapidly acting agents can be given intravenously provided the patient is not already digitalised (page 148). Alternatively, dopamine or dobutamine can be used.
5. *Diuretics*, e.g. frusemide (furosemide) 20–40 mg i.v. Catheterisation of the bladder will usually be required.

Pacemaker

Patients who have complete heart block will have a temporary or permanent pacemaker in place. These should present no problems. It is important, however, to prevent any hypovolaemia or postural hypotension as this may lead to a fall in cardiac output if the pacemaker is on a fixed rate.

It is prudent to have available an alternative method of pacing, such as an oesophageal pacing electrode.

NEUROMUSCULAR DISEASE

Myasthenia Gravis

Myasthenia gravis is a chronic disease thought to be due to a defect in the synthesis or storage of acetylcholine at the nerve ending. Symptoms include progressive muscular weakness and fatigue. One or more muscle groups may be affected; the most common signs are:

1. Eye signs – ptosis, diplopia and blurred vision.
2. Myasthenic facies.
3. Respiratory muscle weakness.

These patients may present problems because of:

1. Altered response to anaesthetic drugs, especially neuromuscular blocking agents.
2. Impaired respiratory function.
3. Labile emotional status with anxiety and depression.
4. Dysrhythmias owing to myocardial involvement.

They are normally receiving maintenance anticholinesterase therapy pre-operatively, but the effects of anaesthesia and surgery may alter requirements, resulting in either myasthenic or cholinergic crises post-operatively.

In view of the complicated management and careful monitoring required, these patients are usually transferred directly to an intensive-care unit after all but the most minor surgery. When they are nursed in the recovery unit, attention must be directed towards:

1. *Maintenance of a clear airway* in the presence of a weak cough reflex and excessive salivation following anticholinesterase therapy.
2. *Maintenance of adequate ventilation* with monitoring of neuromuscular transmission and blood gases, if necessary.
3. *Pain relief.* Small increments of opiates should be given intravenously, with the dose being titrated against the patient's response, if a local anaesthetic block has not been performed.
4. *ECG monitoring and the treatment of arrhythmias.* Respiratory inadequacy occurring post-operatively may be due to either an exacerbation of the myasthenia (myasthenic crisis) or a relative overdose of anticholinesterase (cholinergic crisis). Differentiating between the two can sometimes be made by injecting edrophonium 2–4 mg i.v. If there is no improvement or increased weakness, this indicates a cholinergic crisis. However, differentiation may not be straightforward, and adequate ventilatory support must take precedence over attempts at diagnosis.

Muscular Dystrophy

After general anaesthesia, patients with dystrophia myotonica will be managed in the intensive-care unit with full ventilatory support until normal respiratory function has returned. If they are admitted to the recovery room it must be remembered that they are particularly sensitive to:

1. Suxamethonium (succinylcholine), which may precipitate sustained muscular contractions.
2. Neostigmine.
3. Barbiturates.
4. Opiates.

Paraplegia

1. Frequent changes in posture are required to prevent the formation of skin ulcers at pressure areas. Pressure areas must be adequately padded.
2. Changes in posture should be made slowly to prevent hypotension due to autonomic dysfunction.
3. Stimulation below the level of the cord damage (e.g. bladder distension) may lead to an excessive sympathetic discharge, resulting in hypertension, tachycardia and dysrhythmias.
4. Hypothermia is common, and intravenous and irrigation fluids require warming.
5. Suxamethonium (succinylcholine) may cause hyperkalaemia with subsequent dysrhythmias or even cardiac arrest if given in the weeks or months immediately after the cord has been damaged. Thereafter, it is safe.

LIVER DISEASE

Liver dysfunction can lead to problems in the recovery room because:

1. *Drug metabolism is decreased.* Patients are unable to tolerate normal drug dosages, which must be reduced accordingly. Of special relevance in the recovery situation are:
   (a) Opiates.
   (b) Local anaesthetics, especially amides, e.g. lignocaine (lidocaine).
   (c) Citrate – hypocalcaemia is more likely following blood transfusion.
2. *Plasma cholinesterase may be reduced,* causing prolonged neuromuscular block following suxamethonium (succinylcholine). Assisted ventilation must be continued until adequate muscle power has returned.
3. *Reduction of clotting factors.* Factors V, VII, IX and X, as well as prothrombin and fibrinogen, are synthesised in the liver. Vitamin K deficiency will be a significant contributory factor if there is obstructive jaundice. If

coagulation is impaired, vitamin K (phytonadione) and fresh frozen plasma should be administered. Coagulation studies may be required (see page 106).

4. *Albumin levels are reduced:*
   (a) Diuretics may be required if oedema is significant.
   (b) Drugs bound to albumin, e.g. pancuronium, will be potentiated. This may lead to a prolonged action requiring continued ventilatory assistance.

5. *Renal failure.* In patients with obstructive jaundice, conjugated bilirubin renders the kidneys more sensitive to the effects of hypoxia. To prevent renal failure in these patients, a good urine output must be maintained by adequate hydration and the administration of mannitol.

RENAL DISEASE

Severe renal disease may affect a patient's recovery from anaesthesia because of the presence of:

1. *Uraemia*, which may cause tremor, muscle twitching, convulsions, drowsiness and coma.

2. *Impaired urine production.* With the danger of circulatory overload, intravenous fluids should be restricted. The use of a Metriset will reduce the possibility of accidental infusion of large volumes. Central-venous-pressure measurements will provide a useful guide to requirements. A bladder catheter should be inserted.

3. *Hyperkalaemia*, which may cause a characteristic ECG pattern with high-peaked T waves. If arrhythmias occur, potassium levels may be reduced by insulin and dextrose. In an emergency, calcium may be given to restore the Ca:K ratio.

4. *Acidosis*, which may lead to gasping respirations and require treatment with sodium bicarbonate.

5. *Impaired drug excretion.* Drugs which rely on renal excretion for elimination, such as digoxin and the aminoglycosides, will accumulate, and dosages must be reduced accordingly.

6. *Hypertension.* Blood pressure is frequently raised in this condition so that hypertension occurring post-operatively should be interpreted accordingly.

7. *Anaemia*, which is common. Blood loss must be replaced to maintain the patient's usual low haemoglobin concentration. There is no benefit to be gained by attempting to restore the haemoglobin to what is 'normal' for patients without renal failure.

8. *Arteriovenous shunts.* These must be treated with extreme care to avoid the possibility of damage or clotting. Blood pressure readings should not be taken on the same arm as the shunt. Drugs should not be injected through the

shunt. Intravenous infusions should not be set up in the same arm as the shunt.

ENDOCRINE DISORDERS

Diabetes Mellitus

This is a chronic metabolic disease characterised by hyperglycaemia and glycosuria owing to insulin deficiency or insensitivity. It is associated with small-vessel disease of the kidney, the nervous tissue and the retina.

In the post-operative period, as during anaesthesia, the aim is to prevent:

1. Diabetic ketoacidosis.
2. Hypoglycaemia.
3. Severe fluid loss.

This will be achieved by:

1. *Supportive therapy:*
   (a) Prevention of hypoxia.
   (b) Monitoring of vital signs.
   (c) Assessment of urine output.
2. *Intravenous fluid and electrolyte therapy:*
   (a) 5% dextrose infusion, if the blood glucose level falls below 15 mmol/l.
   (b) Dextrose saline (4% dextrose and 0.18% sodium chloride) is an alternative.
   (c) Regular estimation of the blood glucose may be carried out using Dextrostix and Reflomat. Laboratory estimations of the blood sugar levels at longer intervals should also be undertaken.
   (d) The serum potassium level should be checked and kept within normal limits (3.5–5.5 mmol/l).
3. *Insulin therapy:*
   A wide variety of methods of administering insulin are in use. These include:
   (a) Low-dose intravenous insulin infusion. Between 4 and 12 units/h of soluble insulin with a small amount of Haemaccel to prevent absorption of the insulin through the plastic tubing.
   (b) Regular intramuscular insulin at hourly intervals. Depending on the measured blood sugar level, no insulin may be necessary, and many patients will not require amounts of insulin beyond their normal requirements.
4. *Correction of acidosis:*
   The use of bicarbonate to correct any acidosis is probably unnecessary unless the arterial blood pH is less than 7.10–7.15. Acidosis will usually be corrected

by insulin and intravenous fluid replacement.

5. *Glycosuria:*
   Although a useful sign, levels of glucose in the urine should not now be used to guide management, especially in the early post-operative phase when gross changes in urine osmolality are taking place.

THYROID DISEASE

Hypothyroidism

Hypothyroidism may lead to problems including:

1. Prolonged recovery time owing to decreased metabolic rate and consequent decreased rate of drug metabolism (see page 93).
2. Hypothermia in the post-operative period owing to loss of normal temperature control (see page 100).
3. Tracheal deviation and respiratory obstruction if a goitre is present.
4. Bradycardia (see page 83).

Hyperthyroidism

Problems with patients who have hyperthyroidism include:

1. Labile blood pressure, which may require active management (see page 83).
2. Dysrhythmias (see page 86).
3. Restlessness (see page 96).

The problems of a thyrotoxic crisis have been discussed and the management outlined on page 124.

PHAEOCHROMOCYTOMA

A phaeochromocytoma is a tumour of chromaffin tissue that characteristically produces and excretes excessive amounts of catecholamines. Following incomplete removal, there may be further catecholamine release with:

1. α stimulation causing hypertension (see page 83).
2. β stimulation causing tachycardia (see page 85) or dysrhythmias (see page 87).

If removal has been complete, there may be circulatory collapse requiring treatment with intravenous fluids and vasopressors. Steroid cover may be required if adrenalectomy has been performed.

Patients with phaeochromocytomas require continuous arterial pressure measurement and ECG recording, and should be transferred directly to an intensive-care unit post-operatively.

PORPHYRIA

Porphyria is a rare metabolic disorder characterised by abnormalities of porphyrin metabolism. Serious complications can develop in patients with acute intermittent porphyria, which is exacerbated by the administration of barbiturates, and may therefore present in the recovery room.

Features include:

1. Fever, tachycardia and hypertension.
2. Acute abdominal pain and vomiting.
3. Psychiatric disturbances.
4. Muscle paralysis.
5. Urine which becomes reddish-brown on standing.

An acute attack may require controlled ventilation for a prolonged period, and transfer to an intensive-care unit will be required. Analgesia is best achieved by regional techniques or opiates. It has been recommended that pentazocine should be avoided.

HAEMATOLOGICAL DISEASE

Iron-deficiency Anaemia

Hypoxia must be avoided in patients with iron-deficiency anaemia. There is a reduction in the oxygen content of the blood, though not necessarily in the oxygen tension. The oxyhaemoglobin dissociation curve is shifted to the right. Additional inspired oxygen should be given to these patients post-operatively and the anaemia corrected. Patients with stable chronic anaemias tolerate their reduced haemoglobin concentration well and there is little to be gained by attempting to obtain a 'normal' haemoglobin level.

Haemophilia

Haemophilia is an inherited disorder of coagulation caused by reduced levels of factors VIII (true haemophilia) or IX (Christmas disease). It only occurs in males and results in prolonged bleeding following minor trauma. If such patients require surgery, haematological advice should be sought and replacement clotting factors transfused before the operation. The patient's clotting time should be measured regularly post-operatively and further clotting factors given as required.

Many haemophiliacs are carriers of the Human Immunodeficiency Virus (HIV) because they have been given contaminated clotting factors. Their HIV status should be determined before they come to theatre and appropriate precautions taken. In an emergency, when HIV status is not known, they should be assumed to be HIV antigen positive. Newly diagnosed haemophiliacs are not a high-risk group as the clotting factors currently used are not contaminated with the virus.

Sickle Cell Disease

Sickle cell disease is a recessive hereditary haemolytic anaemia; it is frequently found in patients of African or West Indian descent, and is due to the replacement of normal haemoglobin by abnormal haemoglobin S. In homozygous sickle cell anaemia, 90% of the haemoglobin is of the S variety. In sickle cell trait (the heterozygous state) less than 40% of the haemoglobin is S. These patients usually present no anaesthetic or recovery-room risks.

If the arterial oxygen tension falls below 40 mmHg, the reduced haemoglobin S forms 'tactoids' which distort and rupture the red cells, causing increased plasma viscosity and occlusion of small vessels. The critical level for patients with sickle cell trait is much lower, probably at 20 mmHg. Other variants of sickle cell disease include sickle cell-haemoglobin C disease (SC) and sickle cell-thalassaemia disease. The homozygous patients may have a multiplicity of life-threatening problems due to:

1. Thrombotic lesions in the lungs, kidneys, brain and bones.
2. Hepatosplenomegaly.
3. Shift of the oxyhaemoglobin dissociation curve to the right.
4. Cardiomegaly.

Prevention of sickling is of paramount importance in the recovery room, and management aims to:

1. Prevent hypoxia – administration of oxygen throughout the recovery period.
2. Maintain normothermia.
3. Prevent acidosis – administration of sodium bicarbonate if necessary.
4. Prevent circulatory stasis, e.g. caused by tourniquets or inadequate peripheral perfusion. The prolonged use of a sphygmomanometer cuff for blood-pressure measurement should be avoided. Hypovolaemia and myocardial depression must be prevented.

Post-operative anticoagulation may be required to prevent venous thrombosis and pulmonary emboli.

The signs of a sickle cell crisis are:

1. *Vaso-occlusive:* tissue ischaemia.
2. *Aplastic:* sudden fall in red-cell production leading to weakness and myocardial decompensation.
3. *Sequestration:* usually in the spleen, leading to hypovolaemia and shock.

Deficiency of Clotting Factors

See page 106.

MUSCULOSKELETAL DISEASE

Rheumatoid Arthritis

These patients will often appear chronically ill, undernourished and anaemic. They may need to undergo major joint surgery to correct their restrictive deformities.

Problems in the recovery room are:

1. *Airway:*
   Because of temporo-mandibular joint disease, atlanto-axial subluxation, cervical-spine immobility and laryngeal tissue abnormalities, these patients are often extremely hazardous to intubate and the airway may prove difficult to maintain. A nasopharyngeal airway is often very useful.

2. *Pulmonary function:*
   A restrictive deformity due to costovertebral joint and vertebral disease may be present, as may diffuse interstitial fibrosis. Blood-gas analysis and a lung-function test should be performed pre-operatively. Care should be exercised when opiate analgesics are used so that respiratory depression does not occur.

3. *Bleeding:*
   Chronic anaemia is common and blood loss should be carefully estimated and replaced. Thrombocytopenia may contribute to a coagulopathy.

4. *Steroid therapy:*
   Adequate steroid supplementation is vital both pre- and post-operatively as the patient will be unable to produce adequate endogenous steroid to cover the stress of surgery (see page 147).

5. *Fluid balance:*
   Because of rheumatoid renal disease, intravenous fluid replacement will need caution and urine output may require monitoring.

6. *Transit:*
   If feasible, the patient should be nursed on his bed rather than on a trolley, as it will be more comfortable.

Osteoporosis

Care in lifting or transferring these patients is needed to prevent accidental fractures of their weakened bones.

Ankylosing Spondylitis

In this condition, the vertebral joints gradually fuse so that flexion, extension and rotation of the spine become impossible. It may be difficult to maintain a clear airway in these patients, and the insertion of a nasopharyngeal airway until they are fully conscious will help. The neck may be fixed in a position of flexion and pillows should be adjusted accordingly.

GERIATRIC PATIENTS

The geriatric patient will present many physiological and psychological problems in the recovery room.

1. *Cardiovascular:*
   (a) Decreased myocardial reserve.
   (b) Coronary artery disease.
   (c) Increased susceptibility to dysrhythmias.
   (d) Decreased cardiac output.
   Hypotension, leading to a decrease in oxygen transport, must be avoided, as must hypertension, which may lead to cerebrovascular haemorrhage.

2. *Respiration:*
   (a) Decreased lung compliance.
   (b) Decrease in vital capacity and total lung capacity.
   (c) Increased shunting.
   All these factors will lead to an increased degree of hypoxia and hypercarbia in the geriatric post-operative patient.
   Secretions should be cleared and chest infections prevented by early physiotherapy. The sitting position will aid ventilation although this may prove difficult in the arthritic patient with multiple bony deformities.

3. *Anaemia:*
   These patients are often chronically anaemic and the prevention of respiratory obstruction and hypoxia is thus particularly important.

4. *Renal function:*
   Drug elimination may be slow. Fluid retention and drug accumulation can occur and should be considered when managing the post-operative fluid and analgesic regimen.

5. *Skin care:*
   It is obviously very important to prevent bed sores when the skin is fragile and slow to heal.

6. *Confusion:*
   Every effort should be made to guide these patients through the recovery time without subjecting them to undue anxiety or tension.

7. *Hypothermia:*
   Loss of subcutaneous fat allows heat loss while a reduced muscle mass reduces the value of shivering as a source of heat production.

PREGNANCY

Post-operative recovery-room care for this group of patients includes:

1. Prevention of hypoxia; oxygen should be given.
2. Prevention of hypovolaemia and hypotension.
3. Adequate analgesia and sedation.
4. In late pregnancy the patient should be nursed in the left lateral position, thus preventing the possibility of vena caval obstruction, which may lead to maternal hypotension, and fetal hypoxia and acidosis.

These patients may require reassurance concerning the safety of the unborn child.

MALNOURISHMENT

Special attention must be paid to preventing pressure sores in malnourished patients. Frequent turning will be required if there is a prolonged stay in the recovery unit as trolleys are notoriously firm. Alternatively, the patient may be nursed on a bed. Intramuscular injections are particularly painful as an appropriate muscle mass may be impossible to find. Intravenous or subcutaneous routes are suitable alternatives.

The malnourished are sensitive to many drugs as less drug will be bound to albumin and globulin, and more will be unbound and active. Dosages must be reduced accordingly.

Intravenous feeding may be in progress via a central venous line. Drugs should not be injected into that line nor should it be used for obtaining blood samples.

In severe malnutrition, plasma cholinesterase levels will be low and prolonged neuromuscular block may follow suxamethonium (succinylcholine) administration, so that ventilatory assistance may be required (see page 73).

OBESITY

1. *Airway maintenance* requires careful attention, especially in the patient with a short thick neck.
2. *Ventilation* is impaired by the weight of abdominal contents pressing on the diaphragm, splinting its movements. Atelectasis is common especially after upper abdominal procedures, and results in shunting and an increased alveolar–arterial oxygen pressure difference. The following prove helpful:
   (a) Oxygen by face mask to increase F_iO_2.
   (b) Sitting the patient up to lessen pressure on the diaphragm as soon as consciousness returns.
   (c) Pain relief by epidural or other local anaesthetic block as appropriate.

(d) Physiotherapy to encourage deep breathing.

Progress can be monitored by comparing serial blood gases with pre-operative baseline values. A period of elective ventilation may be required. Extubation should not be performed until ventilatory function is satisfactory.

3. *Deep-vein thrombosis* is more common in the obese patient and early mobilisation should be encouraged. Prophylactic heparinisation is frequently used.

4. *Moving and lifting* patients is difficult and should not be attempted without adequate help.

5. *Venous lines* must be carefully preserved since replacement may be impossible without a cut down.

6. *Blood pressure estimations* by indirect methods are difficult to obtain and the correctly sized cuff must be used (Table 2.3). Hypertension is common in the obese. Arterial cannulation may be the most satisfactory method of obtaining accurate readings.

References and Bibliography

Albert KGMM, Thomas DJB (1979). The management of diabetes during surgery. Br J Anaesth, 51, 693–710.

Aldrete JA, Guerra F (1981). Hematological disease. In: Katz J, Benumof J, Kadis LB (Eds), Anaesthesia and Uncommon Diseases, Saunders, Philadelphia, pp. 313–383.

Bevan DR (1979). Renal function in anaesthesia and surgery. Academic Press, London.

Caldwell TB (1981). Anaesthesia for patients with behavioral and environmental disorders. In: Katz J, Benumof J, Kadis LB (Eds), Anaesthesia and Uncommon Diseases. Saunders, Philadelphia, pp. 672–777.

Chung DC (1982). Anaesthesia in Patients with Ischaemic Heart Disease. Edward Arnold, London.

Davenport H (1986). Anaesthesia in the Elderly. Heinemann, London.

Fisher A, Waterhouse TD, Adams AP (1975). Obesity: its relation to anaesthesia. Anaesthesia, 30, 633–647.

Foex P (1981). Preoperative assessment of the patient with cardiovascular disease. Br J Anaesth, 53, 731–744.

Fox GS, Whalley DG, Bevan DR (1981). Anaesthesia for the morbidly obese: experience with 110 patients. Br J Anaesth, 53, 811–816.

Gareth J (1982). Symposium on anaesthesia and respiratory function. Br J Anaesth, 54, 701–782.

Goldman L, Caldera DL, Nussbaum SR, et al (1977). Multifactorial index of cardiac risk in non-cardiac surgical procedures. N Engl J Med, 297, 845–850.

Gothard JWW (1987). Anaesthesia for Cardiac Surgery and Allied Procedures. Blackwell, Oxford.

Leventhal SR, Orkin FK, Hirsh RA (1980). Prediction for the need for postoperative mechanical ventilation in myasthenia gravis. Anaesthesiology, 53, 26–30.

Marshall AJ (1981). Drug therapy of hypertension and ischaemic heart disease. Br J Anaesth, 53, 697–710.

Prys-Roberts C (1980). The Circulation in Anaesthesia. Blackwell Scientific Publications, Oxford.

Strunin L (1977). The Liver and Anaesthesia. Butterworths, London.

Sykes MK, McNicol MW, Campbell EJM (1976). Respiratory Failure. Blackwells, Oxford.

Taylor TH, Major E (1987). Hazards and Complications of Anaesthesia, Churchill Livingstone, London.

Vickers MD (1982). Medicine for Anaesthetists, Blackwells, Oxford.

Vickers MD, Wood-Smith FG, Stewart HC (1978). Drugs in Anaesthetic Practice, Butterworths, London.

Watkins J, Salo M (1982). Trauma, Stress and Immunity in Anaesthesia and Surgery, Butterworths, London.

Chapter 7
RECOVERY AND DAY SURGERY

Almost 50% of all elective surgery in the UK is now performed on a day-stay basis, facilities ranging from free-standing, purpose-built premises to day wards within a hospital site using dedicated lists in the main theatre suite. It is an efficient way of utilising resources and patient satisfaction can be very high. Since much of the preparation and late recovery of the patient must take place outside the hospital, meticulous organisation is essential and the provision of detailed information for patient, carer and community-health workers is vital.

An increased level of day surgery has been made possible by advances in anaesthesia and surgical techniques, and should not be viewed as 'second best'. Patient safety must never be compromised, which means standards in theatre and recovery room must be equal to those for in-patients. Strict guidelines for selection of patient and procedure should be formulated and observed.

PATIENT SELECTION

Initial referral is usually made from the hospital out-patient department, but can be directly from general practice. It is wise, therefore, to circulate agreed protocols for admission to all those involved in selection. Compliance is particularly important where no pre-admission clinic exists, in order to avoid cancellation on the day, which is both upsetting for the patient and wasteful.

Criteria will vary from unit to unit. Relevant factors are given below:

Social Circumstances

1. The patient should be willing to undergo day surgery.
2. The patient should live, or plan to stay, within a 20 mile radius of the hospital.
3. The patient must be accompanied home (not on public transport) by a responsible adult who should remain available for at least 24 h post-operatively.

4. The home situation should be compatible with the patient's post-operative care, i.e. access to a telephone, adequate bathroom facilities, not too many stairs.

Medical Factors

1. *Age.* An upper age limit is inappropriate. Elderly patients who otherwise satisfy day-surgery criteria should not be denied recovery in familiar surroundings. Although day care is the ideal for paediatric patients, a lower age limit may be necessary in an individual unit because of lack of specialised equipment or staff expertise.
2. *The patient should be generally fit and well.* Any chronic disease, such as hypertension, epilepsy or asthma, should be well controlled.
3. *Diet-controlled diabetics* do well as day cases, but those on insulin or oral hypoglycaemic drugs are better managed as in-patients.
4. *Obesity* can lead to surgical, anaesthetic and recovery problems. The patient should ideally have a Quetelet ratio of less than 30, i.e.

$$\frac{\text{Weight (kg)}}{\text{Height (m)}} \leq 30$$

PROCEDURE SELECTION

A wide range of procedures in many specialties can safely be carried out on a day-stay basis. Several factors should be considered:

1. The procedure should be expected to last less than 1 h.
2. Surgery should not be expected to produce severe post-operative pain or blood loss.
3. The surgery should not render the patient too incapacitated to cope at home.

Examples of Suitable Procedures

General Surgery

Excision of cysts and lipomata
Ligation of varicose veins
Treatment of in-growing toenails
Herniorraphy
Anal dilatation

Orthopaedics

Arthroscopy
Carpal tunnel decompression
Manipulation under anaesthesia
Removal of metalwork
Hand surgery

Urology

Cystoscopy
Vasectomy
Circumcision
Hydrocoele repair

Ear, Nose and Throat [ENT]

Myringotomies
Insertion of grommets
Antral lavage

Reduction of fractured nasal bones
Endoscopies

Pain Clinic Procedures

Chemical sympathectomy
Nerve blocks
I.V. guanethidine blocks

Gynaecology

Termination of pregnancy
Laparoscopy
Dilatation and curettage
Excision of Bartholin's cyst

Oral Surgery

Dental extraction
Apicectomy
Dental conservation in the mentally
handicapped

Paediatric Surgery

Herniotomy
Circumcision
Orchidopexy

PRE-ADMISSION CLINIC

As the scope of day surgery units (DSUs) expands alongside the drive for improved efficiency, there has been an increase in the use of pre-admission clinics. Usually, patients are invited to attend the DSU when their operation date is a few weeks ahead (if waiting lists are short, they can go straight from the out-patient clinic). Here, they are assessed by a senior member of the nursing staff according to protocols agreed for that unit. There are many benefits from such a service:

1. Unsuitable patients can be identified, avoiding cancellation on the day, or pressure to take risks.
2. Any necessary investigations can be performed ahead of time.
3. Patients are able to familiarise themselves with the unit and the staff who will care for them.
4. Detailed information can be given to the patients early so that they can prepare for recovery at home.
5. A convenient date can be booked at this time.
6. There is an opportunity to discuss any fears or questions.

The efficiency of a DSU can be greatly improved by this system; the 'did not attend' rate, cancellation rate and overnight admission rate are all reduced to a minimum. Most importantly, patient satisfaction is very high and anxiety levels decreased.

DOCUMENTATION

Whether or not the patient attends a clinic, clear, *written* information on the general routine of the DSU and specific to the planned procedure should be provided. This should include pre-operative advice on fasting and a warning not to drive or to operate machinery for 24 h post-operatively. It is a good idea to have a standardised questionnaire covering general health, details of escort/ carer, medication list and confirmation of adequate fasting. This can usefully be incorporated into a booklet covering the whole episode such that consent form, admission details, anaesthetic and recovery record, operation note and discharge checklist all stay together and are available to each member of staff involved in the patient's care. Such a chart will enable the recovery nurse to note any areas which may give rise to problems after surgery.

ANAESTHETIC MANAGEMENT

The aim of day-surgery anaesthesia is to relieve anxiety, provide good conditions for surgery and a rapid return to 'street fitness' free from post-operative problems such as pain, drowsiness or nausea and vomiting.

A sympathetic explanation from the anaesthetist can usually replace *pre-medication*, although a small dose of a benzodiazepine drug such as temazepam need not delay discharge. The use of a topical local anaesthetic [EMLA] prior to intravenous cannulation need not be restricted to children and may be very helpful to a nervous, unpremedicated patient.

If *general anaesthesia* is used, agents which are rapidly metabolised and excreted should be used. Propofol is the agent of choice for induction and for infusion as part of a total intravenous technique [TIVA]. *Maintenance* is also satisfactory with a volatile agent and nitrous oxide. Of those available, desflurane produces a more rapid recovery than isoflurane, and sevoflurane has advantages, particularly for paediatrics, where its non-irritant, pleasant smell can facilitate a gaseous induction. Both agents are, however, more expensive than isoflurane and although early recovery is accelerated, time to discharge is not significantly reduced. TIVA has definite advantages for pregnancy termination where uterine bleeding and post-operative nausea and vomiting can be reduced significantly.

Effective intra-operative *analgesia* can be achieved with the ultra-short acting opioids fentanyl or alfentanil. Neither causes undue post-operative somnolence, but analgesia is also short-lived and it is important to provide for *post-operative pain relief* during anaesthesia in order to have a smooth emergence and re-covery. Options for post-operative analgesia include:

1. A non-steroidal anti-inflammatory drug [NSAID] such as ketorolac intra-venously, piroxicam intramuscularly or diclofenac in suppository form.
2. Intravenous or intramuscular tramadol, a longer-acting mixed opioid agonist, without the side-effects of respiratory depression or somnolence.
3. Local anaesthesia. This is an ideal adjunct to general anaesthesia in day surgery. Regional, nerve blocks or local infiltration with long-acting agents such as bupivacaine can give several hours of pain relief without causing

post-operative nausea and vomiting or the other effects of conventional analgesics. It is important not to exceed the maximum recommended dose. Strict discharge criteria must be applied in order to avoid such problems as retention of urine or trauma to the affected area.

If muscle relaxation is required, it is important to avoid the use of suxamethonium if possible. Of course, for safety's sake, it is occasionally essential, but the severe muscle pains following its use are well documented, particularly in the young, fit, ambulant patient so typically treated by day surgery. There are several possible alternatives:

1. Short-acting, non-depolarising muscle relaxants, e.g. mivacurium.
2. Intubation with propofol and alfentanil, e.g. for dental extractions.
3. The use of a laryngeal mask airway often obviates the need for muscle relaxation, e.g. dental extractions.

RECOVERY FROM ANAESTHESIA

Although recovery from anaesthesia for day-case procedures should be rapid and uncomplicated, the same high standards are required as for in-patients. Turnover may be very high on these busy lists and staffing levels should reflect this. Each patient should be positioned appropriately, given oxygen, and have his vital signs monitored and recorded. The Guedel or laryngeal mask airway can be removed carefully once the patient is able to maintain his own airway without support. Day-surgery patients are unlikely to have required an intravenous infusion, surgical drainage or urinary catheter, but nursing staff should have the expertise to cope if necessary. Once they are fully conscious and their condition stable, they can leave the first-stage recovery area and either return to the ward or move on to a specialised area, perhaps equipped with reclining chairs. In this kind of circular system, it is important to avoid disorientation by careful explanation and reassurance.

Many units have introduced a multi-skilled approach whereby nursing staff work in more than one area, for example, recovery and the ward. This broadens understanding, as the same recovery nurse may be responsible for the second stage as well as the ultimate discharge of the patient.

DISCHARGE FROM THE HOSPITAL

Numerous tests have been described that seek to determine when a patient is sufficiently recovered to be discharged. No single test is ideal or a substitute for a careful clinical evaluation.

All patients should be seen after surgery by both surgeon and anaesthetist; responsibility for discharge home can then be taken by nursing staff once the strict criteria are fulfilled:

1. Pulse and blood pressure should be stable and close to admission levels.
2. The patient should be able to dress and care for himself.

3. The patient should have had at least a drink, without nausea or vomiting.
4. The patient should be pain free and provided with suitable oral analgesics to take home, accompanied by written advice on their use with a time for the next dose.
5. The patient should have passed urine.
6. The wound should have been inspected or the dressing checked.
7. Instructions, both verbal and in writing, should be provided, outlining follow-up care, contact phone numbers in case of problems and a warning against driving or operating machinery for 24 h.

Once the checklist is completed and recorded in the notes, the patient can be discharged into the care of a responsible adult who should remain available for 24 h. It is vital that the GP should be aware of the surgery and any prescribed medication. If this information is not faxed or passed on by telephone immediately, then a GP's letter should accompany the patient in case of contact before it can be posted.

There should be no pressure on the patient to leave too early; 2–3 h post-general anaesthesia seems to be optimal, but if a patient feels unwell or the escort is unwilling to accept responsibility, facilities should be available for overnight admission. If the surgery has taken place in free-standing premises, then protocols must be in place for transfer and admission to an in-patient hospital. Hospital hotels can solve problems with the escort/carer, but are not staffed by medical or nursing personnel and therefore the same recovery criteria apply.

Telephone follow-up the next day can be very rewarding for both patient and nursing staff. Many minor problems can be solved by reassurance at this final stage in the recovery process.

PAEDIATRICS

It is generally more appropriate to treat children apart from adults in hospital, where at all possible. Day surgery is considered the best option for about 60% of cases, minimising parent–child separation and reducing disruption in the rest of the family. If whole days cannot be set aside in a DSU for paediatric surgery, then at least accommodation in a specialised bay or individual cubicle is a compromise.

Additional pre-operative instructions are required for paediatric patients:

1. It is useful for the parent or carer to know in advance that he will usually be able to accompany the child to the anaesthetic room and stay until he is asleep.
2. Fasting policies vary, but most anaesthetists are happy to encourage clear fluids until 3 h pre-operatively, as children soon become dehydrated and irritable if starved for long periods.

Management

Topical anaesthesia makes venous cannulation very much easier and premedication rarely necessary. Induction with propofol can cause distressing pain, even when mixed with lignocaine, such that thiopentone may still be the agent of choice. Immediate recovery could take a little longer, but times to discharge are similar.

Local anaesthesia should be employed wherever possible to prevent pain on awakening, and subsequent management is then greatly facilitated. Clear, simple guidelines on recognition and control of pain should be provided with the 'take home' analgesic drugs so that distress can be forestalled. Ibuprofen syrup, given regularly, combined with a paracetamol preparation as required, controls all but the most severe pain.

Both theatre and recovery room must be fully equipped for paediatrics, including warming facilities and specialised instruments.

Recovery will normally be rapid but requires nursing staff experienced with children. It soon becomes second nature to distinguish a child in pain from one who is simply disorientated and needs reuniting with his parent.

POST-ANAESTHETIC COMPLICATIONS

Anaesthetic complications which are seen and treated routinely on an in-patient ward can be considered extremely worrying to a day-stay patient who has returned home. It is very beneficial to spend time warning of the commoner problems which may occur and providing clear details of what to do if symptoms persist.

Most anaesthetic complications are minor and self-limiting, so that explanation and reassurance are often the only treatment necessary.

Pain

Most patients will experience post-operative pain of some degree. It is vital to provide adequate analgesia, not only for the immediate recovery period, but also for the days following discharge, together with a fact sheet on recommended 'over the counter' preparations. Regular audit within a unit should demonstrate whether supplies are 'right first time'. If not, an undue workload may be placed on the community services.

Regional or Local Anaesthesia

Pain or 'pins and needles' will occur as any local anaesthetic block wears off. Backache can be caused by minor local trauma which occurs when epidurals or sympathectomies are performed. Patients should be given oral analgesia as sensation returns.

Hypotension can occur after spinal or epidural blocks as a result of sympathetically mediated vasodilatation. It may manifest itself as dizziness on standing, light-headedness or nausea. Patients should be advised to avoid sudden changes in posture and encouraged to take oral fluids. It is rarely severe enough to warrant treatment with rapid intravenous infusion or sympathomimetic drugs.

Motor blockade can be very worrying if it persists. Patients can be reassured that it rarely lasts longer than 4–6 h. They should also be warned of the potential problem of a partially blocked leg giving way or a partially blocked arm dropping suddenly to their side. The possibility may affect the choice of technique if there are alternatives, for example, a penile block in preference to a caudal, or a local infiltration in preference to a triple block for arthroscopy.

Retention of urine can follow spinal or epidural blocks. It is wise to ensure that patients have passed urine before allowing them home.

General Anaesthesia

Drowsiness is less common and less severe following the relatively brief general anaesthesia required for day surgery than for more complex procedures. However, if severe, it can delay discharge or necessitate admission. Even those who appear to recover quickly will be below par for 24–48 h and must be warned against taking on any responsibilities including household duties as well as driving or operating machinery.

Post-operative nausea and vomiting [PONV] can affect as many as 50% of gynaecology patients, although usually less in other specialities, and is more common as a late complication than in the recovery room. There are many factors involved, such as:

1. Type of anaesthesia.
2. Type and site of surgery.
3. Pain or anxiety.
4. Treatment with opioids.
5. Previous history of PONV or motion sickness.
6. Early mobilisation (hypotension).
7. Female hormones (relationship to menstrual cycle).
8. Rapid recovery.
9. Excessive movement during emergence.

Predictably, with such a multi-factorial symptom, there is no panacea. A rational approach is to prescribe prophylaxis for those who are most at risk and treatment for any who later develope PONV.

Sore throats are traditionally blamed on intubation, but occur almost as frequently in patients who are not intubated. They may be due to breathing dry anaesthetic gases or to the use of Guedel or laryngeal-mask airways. They rarely last longer than 24–48 h and may be alleviated by gargles.

Muscular aches and pains may occur if suxamethonium is used prior to intubation and have been mentioned above. Other non-specific aches and pains may result from lying on the operating table or from the positioning of limbs for surgery. If there is pain or weakness in the distribution of a specific nerve or nerve plexus, the degree of deficit should be carefully recorded and appropriate follow-up management arranged. Most deficits are neuropraxias and will recover spontaneously.

Bruising may occur at injection sites, but needs no specific treatment. If thrombophlebitis occurs, non-steroidal anti-inflammatory agents may help relieve discomfort.

Visual disturbances can be due to the residual effects of general anaesthesia, and regress spontaneously. A sensation of grittiness in the eye will probably be due to corneal drying when the eye-lids have not been closed during anaesthesia. Foreign bodies must be excluded if prompt recovery does not occur.

Most of these problems are annoying rather than dangerous. Much anxiety can be avoided by careful explanation, forewarning and provision of a contact phone number to ring for further advice.

References and Bibliography

Royal College of Surgeons of England (1992). Guidelines for Day Case Surgery. London.

Healy TEJ (Ed) (1990). Anaesthesia for Day Case Surgery. Baillière's Clinical Anaesthesiology, 4(3). Baillière Tindall, London.

Caring for Children in the Health Services (1991). Just for the Day. National Association for the Welfare of Children in Hospital, London.

Wilkinson DJ (1993). Modern Day Surgery in Anaesthesia Review 10 (Ed. Kaufman, L). Churchill Livingstone, London, pp. 163–182.

Chapter 8
MONITORING

All efforts which are made to detect problems early in the vital post-operative recovery period should decrease patient morbidity and mortality. Monitoring is the process whereby systematic observation and subsequent evaluation occur so that actual or potential changes in a patient's physiological state may be quickly recognised. Appropriate treatment can then be initiated. Patient monitoring must, therefore, be a continuous decision-making process. It requires data to be collected and the collector to have sufficient knowledge to interpret and act on those data. Care must be taken, however, to ensure that staff are not submerged by excessive amounts of new data and so miss vital changes in the clinical state of the patient. Observing the patient must remain paramount.

In the recovery area, part of the nurse's role will be to collect and organise data so as to define a particular patient's status. This will often result in situations where the nurse will also interpret data and initiate therapy without referring to a doctor. In other circumstances it will be more appropriate to seek medical advice.

In the early post-operative phase, monitoring is mainly directed towards the detection of complications of recovery from anaesthesia. The degree and sophistication of monitoring will depend on the specific needs of the patient. These needs will be determined by a number of factors including age, anaesthetic risk, metabolic state, pre-existing cardiovascular or respiratory disease, and the often overlooked surgical procedure that has been carried out and the primary disease which made surgery necessary.

Much work has been carried out to determine what is the most appropriate level of monitoring for a given patient, and it appears that three levels of monitoring are necessary:

1. Routine or standard.
2. Advanced or special.
3. Intensive or highly sophisticated.

This last category would be appropriate for those patients who are at high risk of multi-organ failure because of pre-existing disease or surgical intervention. The recovery room should be able to provide either standard or advanced monitoring. Invasive and intensive monitoring are more the domain of intensive care or high-dependancy units.

ASA CLASSIFICATION

The degree of risk for each individual patient must be determined and the appropriate levels of monitoring then provided. Many different techniques of 'risk audit' are now available. Probably the most simple and useful is that proposed by the American Society of Anesthesiologists (ASA) (Table 8.1):

- ASA 1 can be monitored basically.
- ASA 2 and 3 will require a more advanced level of monitoring.
- ASA 4 and 5 will require more advanced monitoring and most probably transfer into an intensive monitoring environment such as the intensive-care unit.

Table 8.1. Physical status classification of the American Society of Anesthesiologists (ASA). Adapted from Anesthesiology, 24, 111 (1963)

Status	Disease state
ASA Class 1	No organic, physiological, biochemical, or psychiatric disturbance
ASA Class 2	Mild to moderate systemic disturbance that may or may not be related to the reason for surgery, e.g. heart disease that only slightly limits physical activity, essential hypertension, diabetes mellitus, anaemia, extremes of age, morbid obesity, chronic bronchitis
ASA Class 3	Severe systemic disturbance that may or may not be related to the reason for surgery, e.g. heart disease that limits activity, poorly controlled essential hypertension, diabetes mellitus with vascular complications, chronic pulmonary disease that limits activity, angina pectoris, history of prior myocardial infarction
ASA Class 4	Severe systemic distubance that is life-threatening with or without surgery, e.g. congestive heart failure, persistent angina pectoris, advanced pulmonary, renal, or hepatic dysfunction
ASA Class 5	Moribund patient who has little chance of survival with or without surgery, e.g. uncontrolled haemorrhage from a ruptured abdominal aneurysm, major cerebral trauma, major pulmonary embolus
Emergency (E)	Any patient in whom an emergency operation is required, e.g. an otherwise healthy 30-year-old female who requires a dilatation and curettage for moderate but persistent haemorrhage (ASA Class 1 E)

ROUTINE MONITORING

This is the usual level of monitoring and can be considered as an extension of routine physical examination which should follow the usual format of such an examination:

1. Inspection.
2. Palpation.
3. Percussion.
4. Auscultation.

For example, one will inspect:

- The skin and nail beds for colour and capillary refill.

- The mucous membranes for colour and, more importantly, for the degree of dryness or moisture.
- The surgical site for swelling or rate of blood loss.
- Movement, to note whether or not it is a purposeful response to a stimulus such as pain or speech.

Palpation will be used to feel for skin temperature, muscle tone, and the volume, rate and regularity of the pulse. *Percussion* may be used to determine the degree of gastric distension or of bladder filling. *Auscultation* is most commonly employed in the measurement of blood pressure with a sphygmomanometer.

RESPIRATORY SYSTEM

The most fundamental observations of respiratory function are:

1. *Colour, central and peripheral.*
2. *Respiratory rate and degree of respiratory effort.* Further respiratory parameters that could be measured in the recovery room include tidal volume (V_t), peak expiratory flow rate (PEFR) and forced expiratory volume (FEV).
3. *Carbon dioxide tension* using:
   (a) Blood gas analysis.
   (b) Transcutaneous CO_2 tension electrodes.
   (c) Capnography.
4. *Oxygen tension* using:
   (a) Blood gas analysis.
   (b) Transcutaneous oxygen tension electrodes.
5. *Oxygen saturation* using:
   (a) A pulse oximeter with the probe on an ear or finger, or, in the case of neonates and infants, across the palm of a hand or the sole of a foot.
   (b) The measurement of mixed venous oxygen saturation in blood taken from a central venous or pulmonary artery catheter.

Post-operative lung ventilation may, on occasions, be required in the recovery room. It is then necessary to have the facility to measure certain aspects of lung mechanics. These will include:

- Expired lung volumes.
- Peak airway pressures.
- Positive and expiratory pressure (PEEP).
- Airway compliance and resistance.

A chest X-ray may often complement the above information especially if a pneumothorax may have occurred following either the insertion of a central venous line, or surgery in the neck or near the diaphragm.

CARDIOVASCULAR SYSTEM

Routine measurement of haemodynamic parameters should include:

1. Heart rate.
2. Blood pressure.
3. Urine output.
4. Temperature.

There should also be facilities to monitor:

1. Electrocardiogram.
2. Blood pressure directly by an arterial line.
3. Central venous pressure.
4. Pulmonary artery pressure.
5. Cardiac output.

Although not routine, the facility to measure these last two parameters should be available and may be useful in the early post-operative management of critically ill patients prior to transfer from the recovery room to the intensive-care unit.

METABOLIC SYSTEMS

The monitoring of these variables will allow for correction of fluid, electrolyte and acid–base abnormalities. It is thus important to measure:

1. Serum electrolytes including sodium, potassium, magnesium and calcium.
2. Blood sugar.
3. Arterial blood pH and bicarbonate.
4. Serum osmolality.
5. Serum urea and creatinine.
6. Urine osmolality.

NEUROLOGICAL SYSTEM

Although neurological monitoring is largely clinically based using the Glasgow Coma Scale (see pages 128–129), it is now possible to use more sophisticated and advanced monitoring techniques in the recovery room. These may be of particular value following carotid artery surgery, neurosurgery and ortho-paedic surgery involving the vertebral column and spinal cord, and are as follows:

- *The electroencephalogram* (EEG). This detects electrical signals from cortical neurones but is often difficult to use as it requires skilled technical interpretation.

- *The cerebral function monitor.* This is a modified and simplified EEG. Three electrodes are placed on the scalp to provide what is known as an *integrated EEG* whereby the voltage generated by EEG signals has been rectified and amplified. Although providing information on the quantity of electrical activity in the brain, this monitor lacks the specificity that is particularly needed following carotid artery surgery.

- *Compressed spectral array.* Using scalp electrodes, this technique presents a histogram of power and frequency change across the range of EEG signals. The EEG frequencies and power are shown in a graphical display on a VDU and changes with time can clearly be seen. Again, this technique is unable to show changes in specific brain areas.

- *Evoked potentials.* These are waveforms generated by the brain in response to specific stimuli. A *somatosensory-evoked potential* (SEP) follows stimulation of a peripheral nerve and may provide information on the functioning of the posterior columns of the cord, the brain stem and cerebral cortex.

- *Brain-stem auditory-evoked potentials* (BAEPs). Auditory signals may be used to test the eighth cranial nerve and provide further information on the functioning of the brain stem and auditory cortex.

- *Visual evoked potentials* (VEPs) use light as the stimulus and the areas assessed will be the occipital cortex, lateral geniculate body and cerebral hemispheres. This path obviously does not include the brain stem.

- *Intracranial pressure* (ICP) monitoring will occasionally be used following neurosurgery and as part of the management of a patient who has had major trauma to the cranium.

SPECIFIC MONITORS

Electrocardiograph (ECG)

An ECG is a graphical representation of variation of cardiac electrical potentials. It is the sum of all the currents flowing through the heart at a given moment and represents the electrical potential of the heart. A systematic approach to analysing the ECG is not beyond the role of recovery-room personnel. If the ECG is routinely monitored in the recovery room, expertise will soon be acquired in recognising the commoner abnormalities.

The standard ECG leads are bipolar, i.e. they record the potential difference between successive pairs of electrodes. They are most useful in the detection of dysrhythmias, conduction blocks, electrolyte disturbances and myocardial ischaemia.

- Lead 1 connects the right arm and left arm electrodes.
- Lead 2 connects the right arm and left leg electrodes.
- Lead 3 connects the left arm and left leg electrodes.

An extension of this bipolar system is the unipolar technique when the three standard leads are used as a common electrode with no potential difference between them. If this is combined with a further active electrode, potential difference between them represents the actual potential. Thus, the unipolar lead system has a neutral electrode formed by the standard leads and an additional electrode termed the 'exploring' electrode. The precordial leads are designated by a letter V plus a numeral corresponding to the location of the electrode on the chest wall. These can be summarised as:

V1. Fourth intercostal space, right sternal edge.
V2. Fourth intercostal space, left sternal edge.
V3. Between V2 and V4.
V4. Fifth intercostal space, mid-clavicular line.
V5. Lateral to V4 in anterior axillary line.
V6. Lateral to V5 in mid-axillary line (see Figure 8.1).

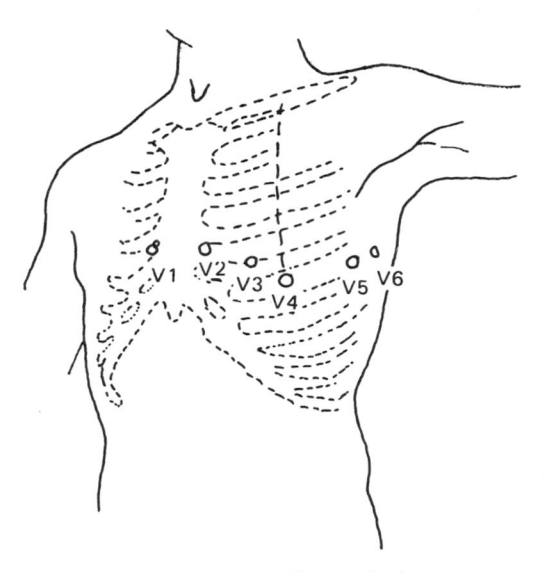

Figure 8.1 Precordial polar leads

The chest leads are useful in interpreting:

- Changes in the rotational axis of the heart.
- Ventricular hypertrophy.
- Bundle branch blocks.
- Antero-septal and lateral myocardial ischaemia.

A further extension of this system is the modified bipolar standard lead, e.g. CM_5. C suggests that the negative electrode is central, M that the positive electrode position has been modified and 5 that the position of this M lead is at V5. Thus the negative right-arm electrode is placed on the sternum, the positive left-arm lead in the V5 position and the ground (or left leg) electrode in its usual left-leg position. This system is particularly useful for monitoring myocardial ischaemia. For monitoring cardiac rhythm, the system MCL_1 is probably of most use (see Figure 8.2).

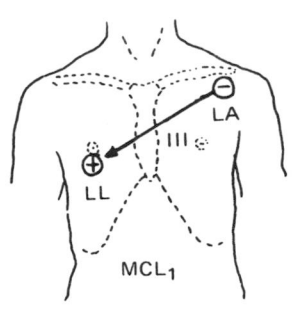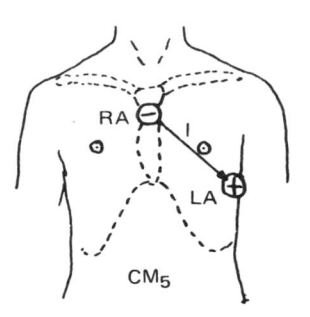

Figure 8.2 Modified bipolar limb-lead systems

ARTERIAL PRESSURE

Arterial pressure may be measured by invasive or non-invasive techniques.

Invasive Methods

These will give continuous-pressure measurements on a beat-to-beat basis and will also allow easy blood sampling for acid–base, blood-gas, electrolyte and haematological measurement and analysis. The site of cannulation is most often the radial, brachial or dorsalis pedis arteries.

Non-invasive Methods

These include the use of Doppler ultrasound transducers and oscillotonometry. Oscillotonometric techniques measure blood pressure and heart rate by means of an inflatable cuff. The cuff inflates to occlude an artery and then begins to deflate in a series of increments. As it does so, the monitor will measure the amplitude of the oscillations induced in the cuff by the movement of the arterial wall. A microprocessor within the monitor will then process and store two consecutive pulsations that have equal amplitude and frequency. At each incremental pressure level, the device stores the cuff pressure, pulsation amplitude and the time between successive heartbeats. Using these variables the monitor notes the pressures when pulsations increase, peak and decrease, and thus determines systolic, mean and diastolic blood pressures and heart rate. Many such devices are now available which will non-invasively record blood pressure and heart rate at predetermined intervals. However, the increased use of microprocessor technology has led to the development of many fully integrated devices which will measure and monitor ECG, blood pressure, invasively and non-invasively, oxygen saturation using an oximeter (see page 181) and carbon dioxide tension using capnography (see page 183). These can either be mounted on a shelf in a recovery bay (Figure 8.3, *overleaf*) or on wheels so that monitoring is uninterrupted during transfer to an ICU (Figure 8.4, *overleaf*).

PULMONARY ARTERY PRESSURE

When patients are critically ill, the measurement of pulmonary artery pressures using a flow-directed balloon-tipped catheter is often indicated. ECG and pressure-wave-form monitoring are needed when a pulmonary artery catheter is being introduced, and full resuscitation equipment should be nearby. The catheter is inserted percutaneously into a central vein and the balloon at its tip inflated. The catheter is carried forward by the blood flow and floats through the right atrium into the right ventricle, and then through the pulmonary artery. Once in the main trunk of the pulmonary artery, it will then float out into the right or left pulmonary artery and will continue until it wedges in a distal branch. The balloon is then deflated and the catheter now measures pulmonary artery pressure. When inflated, the balloon will occlude the distal branch of the pulmonary artery and will measure pulmonary capillary-wedge pressure (PCWP). Wedge pressure reflects transmitted pulmonary venous pressure which approximates left atrial pressure. The left atrial pressure, if the left ventricle is normal, will be the left ventricular end diastolic pressure (LVEDP). The normal PCWP is in the range 6–15 mmHg.

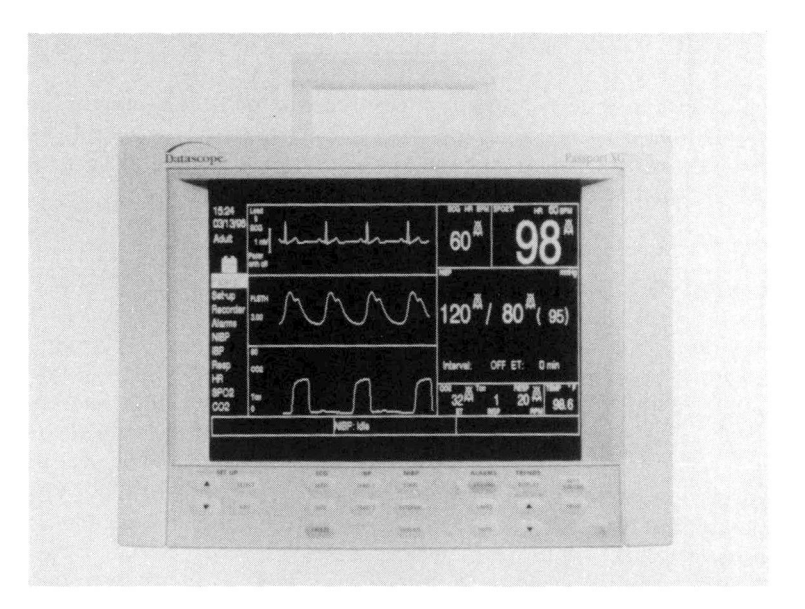

Figure 8.3 Integrated monitoring system; ECG, invasive blood pressure, temperature, oximetry and capnography

It is possible to use a pulmonary artery catheter to measure cardiac output by:

1. The thermodilution technique.
2. The dye dilution technique.

If the thermodilution technique is to be used, a triple lumen catheter is inserted, with a thermistor near its tip and an extra proximal lumen opening into the right atrium. A 10 ml bolus of saline at 0°C is injected into the right atrium. It will mix with blood already there and the transient decrease in blood temperature will be detected by the thermistor lying in the pulmonary artery. From a knowledge of the volume and temperature of the cold saline injected into the right atrium and the subsequent drop in temperature in the pulmonary artery, a cardiac output microprocessor will determine the cardiac output.

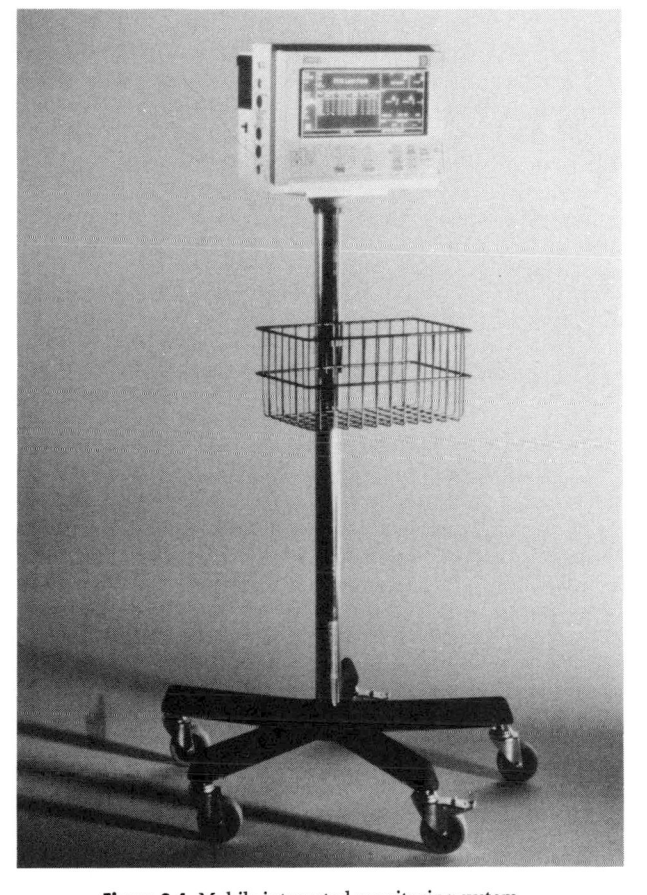

Figure 8.4 Mobile integrated monitoring system

OXYGEN SATURATION

Prior to the availability of the oximeter, the absence of cyanosis was taken as an indication that oxygenation was adequate. Changes in the colour of haemoglobin (Hb) with different degrees of oxygenation have been measured for many years. Recent developments now allow these to be measured accurately and non-invasively utilising the technique of pulse oximetry.

The amount of red light absorbed by Hb varies with its oxygen saturation while the absorption of light of other wavelengths is not altered. Current oximeters send light of several different wavelengths through tissue. The amount of light of all wavelengths received by the detector will depend on the thickness of the tissue and the total amount of Hb present. In addition, the amount of red light received will depend on the degree of Hb oxygen saturation. A microprocessor derives the Hb oxygen saturation from the amount of light detected. The microprocessor is also programmed to record only the saturation of Hb that is in pulsating arteries and to disregard that in non-pulsatile veins. Hence, pulse oximeters display the arterial oxygen saturation and not the total Hb oxygen saturation. The pulse oximeter is designed to be insensitive to haemodynamic changes although extreme hypotension or vasoconstriction may produce a signal too weak for the oximeter to detect. Pulse oximeters are simple to use and non-invasively give continuous information on the degree of arterial oxygenation.

Although they represent a significant advance in non-invasive monitoring, they can be inaccurate in the presence of carboxyhaemoglobin, methaemoglobin and fetal haemoglobin, or in jaundiced patients.

NEUROMUSCULAR BLOCKADE

It may be necessary to monitor neuromuscular blockade to ensure that recovery from muscle relaxants is complete. Many studies have indicated that patients are all too frequently returned to the recovery room partially paralysed. Routine monitoring with a peripheral nerve stimulator makes it possible to achieve precise individual dosing of both muscle relaxants and their antagonists. Some patients have been found to respond in an unpredictable manner to muscle relaxants and therefore monitoring with a peripheral nerve stimulator (PNS) is essential. These include:

1. Patients with a reduced ability to metabolise muscle relaxants, e.g. those with liver and renal disease.
2. Debilitated patients with reduced muscle mass.
3. Patients with neuromuscular disease.
4. Morbidly obese patients.
5. Patients during prolonged surgery.

Whatever particular PNS machine is used, it should have the ability to administer:

1. A single twitch.
2. A tetanic stimulus of 50–100 Hz.
3. Train-of-four (TOF) stimulation.

TOF stimulation is the application of four supramaximal stimuli (2 Hz) at intervals of 0.5 s over a period of 2 s. A patient may be considered to have recovered from the effects of neuromuscular blockers if he shows no evidence of fade on tetanic stimulation and the fourth stimulus in a TOF produces a response that is at least 75% of that of the first. The most commonly stimulated peripheral nerves are the median and ulnar nerves.

CARBON DIOXIDE TENSION

The amount of carbon dioxide in expired air can be measured by a capnometer. This transmits a beam of infra-red light through a chamber into which expired air is constantly drawn. The amount of infra-red light absorbed will depend on the amount of carbon dioxide present. Inspired room air can be assumed to contain no CO_2, whereas a normal end tidal CO_2 will be between 4.5% and 5.5%. The measurement of end tidal CO_2 is useful:

1. As an indicator of the adequacy of ventilation in either the spontaneously breathing or ventilated patient.
2. To monitor the adequacy of cardiac output and blood pressure. This is particularly important following the use of induced hypotension when end tidal CO_2 may fall as less CO_2 is being produced. When normal blood pressure and cardiac output are restored there should be an appropriate rise in end tidal CO_2.
3. As an early warning of a venous air embolism. This results in micro-bubbles of air filling the pulmonary vasculature. This will produce a ventilation/perfusion mismatch with retention of CO_2 in the tissues and a consequent fall in expired CO_2.
4. As a ventilator disconnection alarm. A sudden fall in end tidal CO_2 will suggest that the patient has become disconnected from the ventilator.

References and Bibliography

Blitt CD (1985). Maintaining in Anaesthesia and Critical Care Medicine. Churchill Livingstone, London.
Gravenstein JS, Newbower RS, et al (1983). An Integrated Approach to Monitoring. Butterworths, London.
Lawrence J, Saidman N, Smith T (1984). Maintaining Anaesthesia, 2nd edn. Butterworths, London.
Macintosh R, Mushin WW, Epstein HG (1987). Physics for the Anaesthetist, 4th edn. Blackwells, Oxford.
Sykes MK, Vickers MD, Hull CJ (1981). Principles of Clinical Measurement, 2nd edn. Blackwells, Oxford.
Taylor TH, Major E (1988). Hazards and Complications of Anaesthesia. Churchill Livingstone, London.

Appendix A
DRUGS COMMONLY USED IN THE PACU

British/American Name	Usage and dosage
Adrenaline/epinephrine	Cardiac resuscitation: 1 mg (10 ml 1:10 000) Anaphylaxis: 0.5–1 mg i.m.
Adenosine	3 mg, then 6 mg then 12 mg i.v.
Alfentanil	50–100 mcg/kg then 15 mcg/kg.
Aminophylline	5 mg/kg over 20 min
Amiodarone	5 mg/kg over 20–120 min. Max 1.2 g/24 h
Amoxycillin	250–500 mg tds
Ampicillin	250 mg–1 g qds
Aspirin	Thrombotic prophylaxis: 75–300 mg od
	Analgesia: 300–900 mg 4–6 hrly. Max. 4 g/day
Atenolol	Arrhythmias: 1 mg/min i.v. Max.10 mg or 150 mcg/kg over 20 min
Atracurium	100–300 mcg/kg
Atropine	Cardiac arrest: 3 mg i.v.
	with anticholinesterases 200 mcg/kg
Benzylpenicillin	300–600 mg qds
	50–100 mg/kg in 2–4 doses
Bumetanide	1–2 mg i.v.
Bupivacaine	2 mg/kg in any 4 h period
Buprenorphine	300–600 mcg 6–8 hrly i.v.
	3–6 mcg/kg. Max. 9 mcg/kg
Calcium salts	Calcium gluconate 10% 10 ml (2.25 mmol Ca)
	Calcium chloride 10% 10 ml (6.8 mmol Ca)
Cefuroxime	750 mg–1.5 g i.v. 6–8 hrly
Cephradine	500 mg–1 g i.v. 6 hrly
	50–100 mg/kg in 4 divided doses
	Children: 0.1 mg/kg then 20 mcg/kg
Chlorpheniramine	10–20 mg i.m.
	10–20 mg in 10 ml saline over 1 min i.v.
Chlorpromazine	25 mg i.m.
Cisatracurium	0.15 mg/kg then 30 mcg/kg

British/American Name (continued)	Usage and dosage (continued)
Chlorpromazine (continued)	500 mcg/kg 6–8 hrly i.m.
Co-amoxyclav	1 g tds i.v. slowly
	25 mg/kg tds i.v.
Codeine	30–60 mg i.m. 4 hrly. Max. 240 mg/day
	3 mg/kg in divided doses
Cyclizine	50 mg i.m. or i.v. tds
Dantrolene	1 mg/kg. Rpt to max. of 10 mg/kg
Diamorphine	2.5–5 mg by slow i.v. inj.
Diazepam	10–20 mg i.v. slowly
	100–200 mcg i.v.
Diclofenac	75 mg i.m., 75–150 mg p.r.
	1–3 mg/kg in divided doses
Digoxin	250–500 mcg i.v. over 10–20 min
Dihydrocodeine	50 mg i.m. 4–6 hrly
Disopyramide	2 mg/kg over 5 min i.v. to max. of 120 mg
Dobutamine	2.5–10 mcg/(kg min) by i.v. infusion
Domperidone	30–60 mg p.r. 4–8 hrly
Dopamine	2.5–5 mcg/(kg min) by i.v. infusion
Dopexamine	0.5–6 mcg/(kg min) by i.v. infusion
Doxapram	1–1.5 mg/kg i.v.
Droperidol	2.5–15 mg i.v.
	200–300 mcg/kg
Edrophonium	500–700 mcg/kg i.v.
Enoxaparin	20–40 mg (2000–4000u) i.m.
Enoximone	90 mcg/(kg min) over 10–30 min then infusion at 5–20 mcg/(kg min)
Ephedrine	3–6 mg i.v., 15–30 mg i.m.
Ergometrine	125–250 mcg i.v.
Esmolol	50–200 mcg/(kg min) i.v.
Etomidate	300 mcg/kg
Fentanyl	50–200 mcg then 50 mcg as reqd
	Children: 3–5 mcg/kg then 1 mcg as reqd
Flecainide	2 mg/kg over 10–30 mins then infusion of 1.5 mg/kg for 1h, reducing to 100–250 mcg/kg for 24h. Max. 600 mg/24h
Flucloxacillin	250–1000 mg i.v. qds
	Children under 2 y: quarter adult dose; children 2–10 y: half adult dose
Flumazenil	200 mcg i.v. Repeat to max. of 1 mg
Frusemide/furosemide	20–50 mg at 4 mg/min i.v.
	0.5–1.5 mg/kg
Gallamine	80–120 mg i.v.

British/American Name (continued)	Usage and dosage (continued)
Gallamine (continued)	1.5 mg/kg
Gentamicin	2–5 mg/kg daily in divided doses 8 hrly
Glucagon	0.5–1 mg or unit s.c., i.m. or i.v.
Glucose	For hypoglycaemia: up to 50 ml of 50% soln i.v.
Glycopyrronium	10–15 mcg/kg with 50 mcg/kg of neostigmine
Haloperidol	2–10 mg i.m. every 4–8 h
Heparin	Deep-vein thrombosis or pulmonary embolus: 5–10 000 u i.v. then infusion of 1–2000 u/h i.v. Children: 15–25 u/(kg h) i.v. or 250 u/kg s.c. 12 hrly
Hydralazine	5–10 mg i.v. over 20 min
Hydrocortisone	100–500 mg s.c. or i.v. tds or qds
Hyoscine	200–600 mcg s.c./i.m.
Ibuprofen	1.2–1.8 g daily in 3–4 divided doses. Max. 2.4 g/d 20 mg/kg in divided doses
Isoprenaline	0.5–10 mcg/min i.v.
Isosorbide	2–10 mg/h i.v.
Ketamine	1–4.5 mg/kg i.v. then 10–45 mcg/(kg min) as infusion
Ketorolac	10 mg i.v./i.m. then 10 30 mg 4–6 hrly
Labetalol	50 mg/min. Rpt as reqd. Max. 200 mg
Lignocaine/lidocaine	Arrhythmias: 50–100 mg i.v. then infusion at 4 mg/kg for 30 min, then 2 mg/kg for 2 h, then 1 mg/kg Local anaesthesia: 200 mg of plain soln. 500 mg of adrenaline-containing soln.
Lorazepam	50 mcg/kg i.v. diluted with NaCl
Meptazinol	50–100 mg i.v. 2–4 hrly
Metaraminol	15–100 mg in 500 ml. Dose adjusted to response
Methadone	5–10 mg s.c. or i.m. 6–8 hrly
Methohexitone	50–120 mg Children: 1 mg/kg
Methoxamine	5–10 mg i.v. at 1 mg/min
Metoclopramide	10 mg i.v. slowly tds; < 10 kg: 1 mg b.d.; 10–15 kg: 1 mg tds; 15–20 kg: 2 mg tds; 20–30 kg: 2.5 mg tds; 30–60 kg: 5 mg tds
Metronidazole	500 mg i.v. or 1 g p.r. tds 7.5 mg/kg i.v. or 125–250 mg p.r. tds
Mexiletine	100–250 mg i.v. at 25 mg/min
Midazolam	Sedation: 2.5–7.5 mg i.v. (70 mcg/kg)
Milrinone	50 mcg/kg i.v. then infusion at 0.5 mcg/(kg min)
Mivacurium	70–250 mcg/kg, then 100 mcg/min every 15 min or 8–10 mcg/(kg min) as infusion

British/American Name (continued)	Usage and dosage (continued)
Morphine	10–15 mg/kg i.m. 4 hrly Children: < 1 month: 150 mcg/kg; 1–12 months: 200 mcg/kg; 1–5 yrs: 2.5–5 mg; 6–12 yrs: 5–10 mg
Nalbuphine	10–20 mg 3–6 hrly Children: 300 mcg/kg
Naloxone	100–200 mcg every 2 min i.v./i.m. Children: 10 mcg/kg
Naproxen	500 mg b.d. p.o./p.r.
Nefopam	60–90 mg tds p.o.
Neostigmine	50–70 mcg/kg with or after atropine
Nitroprusside	0.3 mcg/(kg min) titrated to effect
Noradrenaline/norepinephrine	80 mcg/ml at 0.16–0.33 ml/min according to response
Ondansetron	4–8 mg t.d.s.
Oxytocin	5 u i.v. post-Caesarean section 5–20 u by slow i.v. infusion for postpartum haemorrhage
Pancuronium	50–100 mcg/kg, then 10–20 mcg/kg as required
Papaveretum	7.7–15.4 mg i.m. 4 hrly
Paracetamol/acetaminophen	500 mg–1 g 4–6 hrly. Max. 4g/day Children: 10 mg/kg
Pentazocine	30–60 mg 3–4 hrly Children: 0.5–1 mg/kg
Perphenazine	4 mg t.d.s. Max. 24 mg/day. Not recommended for children
Pethidine/meperidine	1 mg/kg 3–4 hrly
Phenazocine	5 mg p.o. 4–6 hrly
Phenobarbitone/phenobarbital	50–200 mg q.d.s. i.m./i.v.
Phenoperidine	1 mg/i.v. then 500 mcg–1 mg every 40–60 min Children: 100–150 mcg/kg
Phenoxybenzamine	1 mg/kg in 200 ml saline over 2 h
Phentolamine	2.5 mg as reqd.
Phenylephrine	100–500 mcg i.v. **N.B. Must be diluted as presented as 10 mg/ml solution**
Phenytoin	15 mg/kg at a rate not exceeding 50 mg/min Children: 15 mg/kg at a rate of 1–3 mg/(kg min)
Potassium chloride	1.5 g (20 mmol) over 2–3 h
Prilocaine	400 mg is used alone. 600 mg is used with adrenaline/felypressin
Procainamide	100 mg at 50 mg/min. Max. 1 g
Prochlorperazine	12.5 mg i.m. or 25 mg p.r. 6 hrly. Not recommended for children
Promethazine	25–50 mg. Max 100 mg
Propofol	2–2.5 mg/kg at 20–40 mg every 10 s
Propranolol	1 mg/min. Max. 10 mg

British/American Name (continued)	Usage and dosage (continued)
Protamine	1 mg neutralises 100 u heparin. Max. 50 mg
Ranitidine	150 mg p.o. or 50 mg i.m./i.v. 6–8 hrly
Rocuronium	600 mcg/kg at induction, then 150 mcg/kg
Salbutamol	500 mcg s.c./i.m. 250 mcg i.v.
Spironolactone	100–200 mg daily
Streptokinase	250 000 u over 60 min, then 100 000 u every hour
	Myocardial infarction: 1 500 000 u over 60 min, then aspirin 150 mg daily
Suxamethonium	600 mcg/kg
	Children: 1–2 mg/kg
Temazepam	20–40 mg p.o.
	Children 1 mg/kg
Thiopentone/thiopental	100–150 mg i.v. up to 4 mg/kg
	Children: 2–7 mg/kg
Tranexamic acid	0.5–1 g t.d.s.
Trimeprazine	2 mg/kg p.o.
Trimetaphan	3–4 mg/min according to response
Valproate	400–800 mg (up to 10 mg/kg) i.v.
	Children: 20–30 mg/kg daily
Vasopressin	20 u over 15 min
Vecuronium	60–100 mcg/kg, then 20–30 mcg/kg as reqd
	Children: 10–20 mcg/kg
Verapamil	5–10 mg i.v. over 2–3 min

Appendix B
TRANSLATIONS OF STANDARD RECOVERY PHRASES

English	Open your mouth	Breathe deeply	Have you pain?	Your operation went well	Time to wake up
Arabic	Iftah fammak	Nafass shadeed	Fee alum?	Ama lia nagahet	Iss ha
Dutch	Open uw mond	Diep ademhalen	Heeft u pijn?	Alles is goed	Wakker worden
French	Ouvrez la bouche	Respirez pro-fondément	Est-ce que vous avez mal?	Votre opération s'est bien passée	Reveillez-vous
German	Mund offnen	Tief atmen	Tut es weh?	Die Opera-tion ist gelungen	Aufwachen
Greek	Aneekse to stoma su	Anapnevse vathia	Echees pono?	El enhirissi sou pigay kala	Ohra na ksipnisis
Hindi/Urdu	Apna moonh kholiay	Lamba sans lee-jaye	Apko kaheen darad hay?	Apka aperation theek ho gayahay	Abb jaag jao
Italian	Aprite la bocca	Respirare profonda-mente	Avete dolore?	La vostra operazione e andata bene	E ora di svegliarvi
Japanese	Kuchi-o aitè	Shinkokyu-o shittay	Itami-ga arimasu-ka?	Shujutsu-wa seiko desu	May-o aitè
Portuguese	Abra la boca	Respire fundo	Esta com dor?	A operacao foi bem	Acorde!
Spanish	Abra la boca	Respire pro-fondamente	Tienes dolor?	Tu operacion a salido buen	Despiertese
Swedish	Oeppna munnen	Andas djupt	Har du Värk?	Din opera-tion gick bra	Tid att vakna

INDEX